My Wonderful Nightmare

My Wonderful Nightmare

Spiritual Journals Inspired by Cancer

Erin Higgins
&
Alma Lightbody

Order this book online at www.trafford.com
or email orders@trafford.com

Most Trafford titles are also available at major online book retailers.

Cover art by Nubia Gala Siebert "Garden of Surprises II" collection of Sylvia Sierra

Printed in the United States of America.

ISBN: 978-1-4251-8725-5 (sc)
ISBN: 978-1-4907-5346-1 (e)

Trafford rev. 12/30/2014

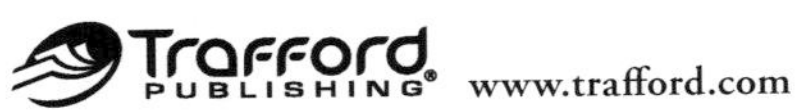

www.trafford.com

North America & international
toll-free: 1 888 232 4444 (USA & Canada)
fax: 812 355 4082

To: Mom, Dad, Lara, Sean

and

All those who were part of my growth

"In opening this book, it is like opening my heart please treat it with a kindly respect for life – yours and mine."

~ Erin

Table of Contents

Acknowledgements:

Erin made numerous notes from books she read, including specific phrases and words that were meaningful to her. She didn't always record where they came from.

I used many of these sentences and quotes throughout the book and would like to acknowledge and thank all the authors who wrote them. Their presence and meaning is a beautiful part of Erin's story.

Other Acknowledgements:

Sylvia Taylor	- Literary Consultant
Jodie Gastel	- Layout and Format
Julie Salisbury	- Inspire-A-Book
Nubia Gala Siebert	- Cover Art

and to

Family and friends that provided helpful proofing and input.

INTRODUCTION

By Alma Lightbody

"If you don't have a test, you don't have a testimony"

Erin shares a legacy of inspirational lessons as she uses the "strength of her soul in the face of tragedy" to find and fulfill her purpose in life.

This book is not for the lighthearted individual who is looking for a simple, happy story. It is for those who are willing to look at the deeper side of life and have the courage to travel with Erin as she steps into the underworld. She is willing to share this journey, and invites you to take a step into the depth of your own soul as you journey with her. As an individual, a patient or a caregiver, here is your opportunity to understand what transpires as the soul exposes itself and prepares to transcend.

As she grew up, Erin was always a caregiver. In the midst of her parent's divorce she took the Mother-Hen role for her siblings very seriously and helped them through uncertain times. Her own marriage was fraught with dominance and control issues and Erin continued with her focus of caregiver to try to make things work. Finally she broke loose to find her own voice and look for the person she wanted to be – independent and in charge of herself. With this goal in mind she left Toronto and returned home to the west coast to be close to family and friends.

The move allowed Erin to find the job of her dreams; Sales Manager for Monk McQueen's Restaurant. She loved working with people, organizing events and being in the social limelight. This was her time to shine and she thrived on it.

Erin's life to date had been a Garden-of-Surprises and already another was waiting around the corner. During her divorce, her life was unsettled and her health in question. Her body messages were subtle and not picked up by the doctors she saw so the internal rumblings continued brewing in her body. Now back in Vancouver, her symptoms continued to progress and she decided to find a doctor that would truly listen to her. She demanded extensive investigation and exploratory surgery. The CAT scan uncovered several unusual areas of growth in her uterus and she was told they could be fibroids or cancer tumours. The surgery was booked immediately.

Erin awoke from this whirlwind of investigation and subsequent surgery to a diagnosis of ovarian cancer. The doctors had proceeded with a full hysterectomy to remove three tumours but some cancer still remained and could only be dealt with through the use of heavy chemotherapy. This diagnosis was a surprise to the doctors because it was such a young age for ovarian cancer to occur. It was easily missed at earlier stages because the messages were mixed and subtle.

Prior to surgery Erin had an inner knowing something was wrong that would change her life-direction. She was a fighter and reset her focus as her perception of who she was began to change once more. The 'Picture Puzzle' she had been living was broken and in chaos. Erin was on a new journey, destination unknown, but somewhere within there was a glimmering light focused on Purpose. Who am I? Why me? Why now? What am I to learn from this?

From the very beginning of this life-changing event Erin wrote about her thoughts and feelings in her journals and often referred to how the value of what she was learning could help others. She said "I believe that my purpose in life is to have this cancer, beat this cancer and teach others with this cross-to-bear how to get through it. That is why I promise to record my thoughts, emotions and physical feelings throughout this challenge. I believe that my experience will serve a purpose to someone I know or will know."

My husband, Mack and I had known Erin's father and his wife Sylvia for a long time but only knew of his children through conversation. Brian stayed at our house when he came to Vancouver to see Erin in the hospital and talked to us about her surgery and diagnosis. With background as an Energy Worker, I said I would be happy to work with Erin if she was interested in such therapy, and she was.

"Energy Work" is our oldest form of healing and has been used in various therapeutic forms across time and cultures. The body's seven invisible energy centres, called chakras that flow up the body from tailbone to crown, have been found as pictures on cave walls, and structures going back thousands and thousands of years. Working with these energy centres for healing is a gentle way of providing comfort, relieving pain, creating balance and helping the mind, body, and soul return to its natural harmonious state. I began to study and practice energy healing twenty years ago and have been involved with several teachers and modalities. The practice Erin refers to exclusively in her journals is called Healing Touch and for simplicity I will use the same terminology.

Everything in the world, including our body is made up of energy waves. We can see our physical body but most of us cannot see the energy system that flows through and around it. As an Energy Worker I am trained to sense and feel this energy and channel and guide pure Universal and Earth energy into the patient to help heal a depleted or damaged area of the body. Normally a healthy body is able to do this work on its own. It's just as simple as breathing and happens without conscious awareness. Bodies that have been traumatized by accidents, illness, surgery, abuse, and so on need help to rebuild and balance their energy fields. That is where an Energy Worker can help.

Erin's most damaged energy centre was the second chakra in the belly that is connected with the uterus/ovaries – a sensitive and hormone-driven centre. It is a perfect place to stuff and hold on to emotional and stressful issues. When energy doesn't flow well through a compromised centre it also limits the flow of energy to other parts of the body so other chakras have to work harder to maintain the body systems. These limitations, along with stressors like surgery and chemotherapy, deplete and drain all the energy systems. Erin and I worked routinely at supplementing and supporting her damaged second chakra as well as her complete energetic field with channeled energy. It was a joy for me to be able to place my hands on her and bring comfort and healing to her mentally and physically. Erin was an excellent student and advocate of this work and practiced it on her own between sessions.

In some of the treatments, along with Healing Touch, I included intervention at a deeper, cellular and soul level to enable Erin to purge and release buried issues that created blockages in her weakened energy centres. One of the techniques I use in such a case is to carefully listen to the dialogue of the patient prior to treatment. I then use that information and craft-it-as-a-question to reflect back to the patient while they are in a relaxed and altered state on the therapy table. The answer to what they need to know is already within them but in our western society we are not taught how to access it easily. Using this technique enhances that opportunity.

Erin just loved it when an intuitive awareness surfaced for her. She would burst out with "Where did that come from?" Her findings created a lot of dialogue and fun between us and because her amazement and excitement were contagious, we would often laugh at the experience.

When a buried issue is exposed it needs to be acknowledged then with clear intent easily released, without having to relive the incident.

We can learn from a very simple technique that wild animals use to release stressful issues. When they encounter a fearful event or interaction they experience it fully, and when it's over, shake their body from head to tail for a few minutes. Animals release the experience and naturally adjust their nervous and energetic systems to their normal state. Unfortunately we, as humans, have lost our ability to quickly pull ourselves out of a profound response and release the associated feelings. Instead, we retain all events in cell memory and it burdens us, diminishes our energy, and sometimes makes us ill. The 'animal reaction' is a small but powerful example of the value of releasing things that do not serve us.

Erin's experience with cancer inspired her to find therapeutic tools to facilitate a depth of clearing and shedding that would enable her to find her Purpose and heal her Soul. The tools she chose where powerful, visual, and cathartic but served her journey well. They were Journal Writing, Healing Touch, and Diet Detoxification, amidst love and support from family and friends. All were a form of purging, clearing, letting go, and connecting with God.

I first met Erin in the hospital a couple of days after her surgery. Here was a beautiful and bubbly thirty-one year-old woman and it was hard to believe what she had just gone through. We hit it off immediately and even though she had never experienced energy work before she was very open and receptive to the concept and to the work itself.

Energy treatments and therapy were a major part of our relationship throughout Erin's journey. She got excited about what she experienced and learned and was anxious to share these findings with others. A subject very important to her was about 'listening' to your body.

"We've never been taught to listen to our body and it's tragic. I somehow knew the results of my surgery before they told me. If I had been more in tune with my body I would have known earlier. I hadn't paid attention and didn't know how. If your body is telling you something is not right, ask for tests, look into it and don't be brushed off. Don't let doctors tell you nothing is wrong. Be aggressive with them – take control. When things bothered me over two years ago it could have made a difference to my outcome if they had been dealt with then."

In addition to writing daily journal entries, Erin talked about using them to create a book about her story. As we discussed this concept further it was agreed I would help compile the information from her journals to share her insights and teachings. Based on this discussion, she said, "I'm leaning towards having my journals tell my story – honest, emotional, real, good advice. I think deep down, that is what is needed out there. Each chapter should take the reader chronologically through my journey."

The story told from these journals takes us on a courageous and inspiring journey as Erin finds her way through the maze of conventional and alternative medicines and the myriad of decisions she is faced with as she fights for her life. She uses her writing as a teaching tool sharing genuine feelings and experiences as she speaks directly to you, the reader.

Her words are informative and fun in some places but also deeper, sadder and more painful than the picture she often showed to family and friends. Writing her thoughts in this way allowed her journals to be her deepest confidant – someone she could talk to, tell all to. They were an outlet for her honest feelings and emotions about living, dying, and spirituality. She says about journaling "The writing is therapeutic and it clarifies things in the mind that the subconscious speaks to. It's a way of venting, of celebrating, and of grieving personal issues. It's been paramount to my healing."

Although, in the end, Erin's story is not about ultimate curing and survival, she began her journals with a focus on how she could help herself and others to "beat the cancer." Even though her outcome changed, her advice and insights are still powerful and speak to all of us. She talks about not being a victim, being an active participant in all decision-making, listening to body messages, using alternative therapies, living in the moment, the value of love, laughing a lot, and many more powerful insights. Erin always brought a genuine honesty and reality to the forefront and continued to write about the depth of her emotions even as her illness became more difficult to cope with. Erin is willing to share these innermost feelings with us and let the "words fall were they may."

In the last few months of her life, Erin came to the realization that spiritual healing may occur but her body would not survive. Her father expressed the same awareness, "I've never been faced with such a juxtaposed position. The spirit was something other than her body. The body is only a vehicle. It was an illumination for me that our body is not us – she was something other than her body."

Such a profound awakening paves the way for the soul to find its way home easily and peacefully. It also helps those caregivers who carry the grief of the loss, to honour this beautiful transcendence of the soul.

PART I

Journals:

by Erin Higgins

"For Erin, cancer was a vehicle for her to teach others. She changed everyone around her."

~ Lara Higgins

CHAPTER 1

The Challenge

"Let's take another sip"
~ Erin Higgins

When the student is ready – the teacher will appear.

For Erin, the teacher was cancer and for the reader, the teacher is Erin.

The journal writings throughout this book are excerpts from Erin's daily entries about her journey with cancer from February 9, 1998 to August 25, 2000. You will see how she writes directly to you, the reader. As you journey with her, look for the underlying messages that stand out from the literal day-to-day experiences. Some are pull-outs in bold but there are many other insights within her words. Dialogue in 'italics' is from co-author, Alma Lightbody

"As you read these words, please do so with an open mind and heart. There may be some part of my journey that can help you."
~ Erin

February 9, 1998

This date will be ingrained in my memory forever. It was a Monday, seemingly like any other Monday except I was going in for surgery. We were hoping it was fibroids, large and growing quickly. I had felt an incredible calm, very peaceful spirit, the entire weekend before going in. Monday morning was like any other except that I was absolutely starving from the fasting on Saturday and Sunday. I had full confidence in my surgeons. I say surgeons (plural) because no one could figure out what this was.

The ultrasound and MRI were inconclusive. My ovarian cancer marker was slightly elevated but "non-specific."

Walking up the road, arm in arm, with Dad and his wife Sylvia, a street woman whom I had seen around Vancouver passed us on the other side of the street. She was playing with her dog. She stopped, looked right at me and yelled across the street:

> "Don't worry – everything is going to be okay. Just take it one day at a time."

Little did I know at the time how prophetic this statement would be. I think back on it now and get goose bumps. I believe that God sends his messages to us in all kinds of ways – from his lips, to her lips, to my ears.

February 10, 1998 – day after surgery

My surgeons came in at 8:15 am and told me that I had had a hysterectomy and had some cancer remaining. I would recover in hospital then start Chemotherapy (chemo). My family was there and I think I held up better than they did. But again, for some reason, none of this shocked me. I felt calm, at peace with myself and was completely accepting of this latest challenge in my life. I had some depression and some feelings of loss for the children I would never have but I had decided before the surgery, that I wanted my surgeons to do whatever they had to do to make me well.

February 11, 1998

I am healing in leaps and bounds! The catheter came out today. I got up to go to the bathroom tonight. The visitors, cards, and flowers are in abundance. I am truly amazed at the amount of support I have. I am so lucky!

This afternoon was brutal. Dr. M. came in and dropped what seemed like a death sentence on me. Dad and I cried, and then I asked him to leave me alone for awhile. The doctor spoke about the amount of chemo I would need and said I wouldn't be able to work. I was devastated! She had a horrible bedside manner.

Looking back on it I can now see that she did have some positive things to say. My age, my strength, and the fact they had removed the tumours were working in my favour but at the time I was very sad. Dad and Sylvia told Mom about the plan when she arrived and I heard her completely break down in the hallway. She knew how important it was for me to be able to go back to work.

Dr. H. came in later that night and re-explained things. It's amazing what a difference a little positive feedback can do with the same message. She eased my mind, somewhat.

February 12, 1998

The first time I met with Alma, a holistic therapist, was while I was still in the hospital. My stomach was very sore from the surgery. She was able to 'pull' the hurt away – literally and physically I felt less pain. This was the first time I had experienced energy healing and balancing. I believe that if she and I continue working together with the energy it will be very helpful. The power of mind over body is absolute.

February 13, 1998

Friday the 13th is usually one of my better days and today was no exception. There were, as always, lots of people visiting today. I have been amazed at the love and support that has walked into this room. I honestly did not know that I had so many people that thought so highly of me! I guess what goes around comes around. It really does pay to be a good friend in good times – the support it then lends in bad times is priceless.

My sister Lara, so innocently, told me today that I couldn't have a shower because the staples in my incision would rust. Everyone in the room just broke out in laughter and we couldn't stop. I had to hold my stomach. That week in the hospital we all laughed a lot. Sometimes it was tiring but also very exhilarating.

February 14, 1998

Happy Valentines Day! I'm so happy today. All my friends came over to be here when I got home from the hospital. There were seven of us: Lara, Kathy, Jen, Phillipa, Christine, Kim and myself standing around my kitchen counter with a glass of wine to celebrate with a toast to health. I put my glass down, thought about it, then raised my glass again and said "Let's take another sip."

In their deep discussions that day, Erin told her friends, "I may be the best person to deal with this illness because I have the strength that all of you can learn from. I can be a teacher."

> *This statement is a simple comment but subtly sets the agenda for her continued commitment to share what she learns with others.*

February 15 to February 21, 1998

I'm feeling more and more nervous about Monday – my first chemo treatment. I'm not afraid of it. Actually, I welcome it. As sick as it will make me feel it represents healing. How ironic that I have to make myself sick to get better!

The past two weeks since I got home have progressed very well. I thank God every day for my strength and a new day. I do take all of this one day at a time and enjoy every minute of every day. I feel strong.

My job at Monk McQueen's Restaurant is the dream job I had been waiting for. They have been so understanding and are letting me work on my own schedule. I have been back at work, off and on, since twelve days after surgery. Work has been extremely therapeutic for me. The support system there is amazing. I know that I need my work to get me through this. I will work from home and go into work when I can. I am counting on eight days after chemo of feeling awful but it is my goal to not let it go further than that. I AM DETERMINED NOT TO LET CHEMO STOP MY LIFE FOR SIX MONTHS. I will be out and about as much as possible.

I thank God every day for my strength and a new day. I do take all of this one day at a time and enjoy every minute of every day. I feel strong.

I can't think of anything but the chemo. It is such a dreaded word. I went for lunch with a cancer survivor today. Unfortunately, she couldn't really tell me much about how I will feel. She said two things that stick in my mind.

1. You don't realize how sick you are with cancer until you start the chemo treatments – then it really hits home that if treatments make you feel this bad, the disease must be horrific!
2. The steroids make your mind race – it takes you places that you really don't want to go but you have to. Just let it happen – eventually it fades.

These two points really hit home. It makes me worry more about chemo. Then I adjust my thinking and remember that this is going to be good for me in the end. BRING IT ON!

In six months I will have willed the cells DEAD with the help of chemo, strong will, and a lot of visualization during the treatments. I want to be alone when each treatment is administered because this is my visualization time.

I strongly believe that what you will to happen can happen. I can see the cells dying and being excreted in urine or coughs or bowel movements. Either way they WILL DIE because I refuse to have them in my body. They lived there for a while when I was unaware but now that I know about them their squatter's rights have officially been revoked. I am EVICTING them from their home. Since they will not leave peacefully I am forced to bring in an army of soldiers. I have consulted with my war commanders (Dr. H. & Dr. S.) and collectively we have decided that Battalions, Topotecom, Cisplatin and Taxol are the strongest and will be the most effective in killing these intruders. Tomorrow is 'D'day boys, so prepare to die – anything less than this is unacceptable. Prepare to be bombarded for six months – your death is inevitable.

February 24, 1998

Alma came to see me today for a Healing Touch session. I find these to be very powerful and relaxing. I really feel a difference with them. I think my body accepts the energy and works well with it. She explained that our emotional centre is in our abdomen. I believe my last few years of emotional trauma may have had an effect on my body. I will teach that one day, to all who will listen. YOU MUST DEAL WITH YOUR EMOTIONS TO COMPLETION – or it can have a negative – possibly lasting effect on you physically. I will continue to see Alma before and

I believe my last few years of emotional trauma may have had an effect on my body. I will teach that one day, to all who will listen.

after every chemo treatment. I believe in what she does and will practice it on my own.

February 25 to March 6, 1998

My spirituality heightens with every day. I feel like I am on a different plane from everyone else. I find it very difficult to sit with a group of people and talk about daily things.

My spirituality heightens with every day. I feel like I am on a different plane from everyone else. I find it very difficult to sit with a group of people and talk about daily things.

I find that unless the conversation is very deep, spiritual, or significant I can't follow it. I can no longer chit-chat. My mind continues to wonder to the cancer, to the treatments and to what more I can be doing about it.

Everything is different now.
Everything smells different, looks different and feels different. Life is very spiritual now – forever changed by a horrible disease – but I appreciate it so much. I really enjoy time alone now, more than ever. It seems to be very important to me. I can't wait to get home and write in my journal or read or study. Television is now a waste of time that I can rarely enjoy. Life is very short, too short to let a single minute pass that is not meaningful. This disease has affected everything around me this way. Lives are forever changed by this.

Life is very short, too short to let a single minute pass that is not meaningful. This disease has affected everything around me this way. Lives are forever changed by this.

The little things don't matter any more. I went to return a shirt that I bought a month ago now. The sales lady told me that there was nothing she could do because I had bought it on sale. The shirt is torn! She still would not refund my money. I didn't care! I tried, she said no and I said thanks anyway and left. Two months ago I would have jumped up and down, yelled and fussed until I got something from her. Now, it's just not worth giving away my energy for. It's just not important enough. DON'T SWEAT THE SMALL STUFF!

I often wonder how long I have had cancer. How long have I been living with this disease? Did I have it when I went to Australia? Was it there when I was married? Is it the reason that I was not getting pregnant for the year that we tried? If it had been caught earlier would I have needed a hysterectomy? I strongly believe that if I had been diagnosed years ago, even one year ago, I would not have been able to handle it. I even would go so far as to question my ability to survive it back then.

I believe that my purpose in this life is to have this cancer, beat this cancer and teach those around me about life, struggle, strength, and insight.

I was very weak spiritually and emotionally in my twenties. I believe that this disease was 'to be' for me from the time I was born. I believe that it waited until now to progress because this is the one time in my life that I can handle it.

I believe that my purpose in this life is to have this cancer, beat this cancer and teach those around me about life, struggle, strength, and insight. Maybe even to teach others with this cross-to-bear how to get through it. That is why I promise to record my thoughts and physical feelings throughout this challenge. I believe that my experience will serve a purpose to someone I know or will know.

I am truly not afraid of this long road ahead of me. It will be the biggest challenge of my life to date. It will be long and very difficult. I have the most incredible support system I could ask for and a stubborn streak in me to get me through it. I pray for healing and compassion from above.

I have cut all of my hair off – short! My hair was to my mid-back and when I found out that the treatments would cause me to lose my hair I decided to cut it short to decrease the trauma of going bald. I LOVE my hair short! I would suggest to anyone beginning chemo to do this.

Laughter is very important in healing. I'm lucky to have a family and friends who laugh a lot. This will be important to my healing – I feel that already. I know the power of laughter is amazing!

There are enough traumas in this disease – don't lose your hair when it's long. I will also shave my head when my hair begins to fall out. Why put yourself through the hair on the pillow, the clumps coming out in your hand – just shave it! I have bought several funky hats – might as well look good if you are bald!

I also went last week to be fitted for my wig. It will look like my hair now, same length and colour.

I believe the better you look when you are sick, the better you feel. I want to make this as comfortable as possible for me to be out and about during chemo. To me, the more normal I look the more normal I will feel. It is very important to me to maintain as much normalcy in life as possible and to do what ever I can do to continue enjoying and getting as much out of everyday as possible.

Laughter is very important in healing. I'm lucky to have a family and friends who laugh a lot. This will be important to my healing – I feel that already. I know the power of laughter is amazing! It healed me after the hysterectomy in incredible time. I can remember days in the hospital when I would have some pain – everyone would be there and inevitably all would laugh and laugh from stories being told or the personalities in the room. It would hurt like hell to laugh with an incision like mine but it was great all at the same time! True, honest, deep laughter has healing powers in itself.

My friends are coming to my first chemo with Mom and Dad tomorrow morning. Thank you for the support you guys! I love you all very much! You are all an integral part of my healing.

With my friends and family around me I will get through this chemo and ultimately, the cancer! I believe this in my heart and soul – God willing and I believe he is. BRING IT ON!!! YOU CANCER CELLS, WILL BEGIN TO DIE!!!

March 8, 1998

I saw Alma again today. I have been there three times now and seem to get very consistent results – that being: more energy and a sense of purity, by getting rid of toxins in my body. I usually have very low energy when I get there.

I feel zapped. From the first time I met with her I have been able to physically feel the energy transference. I can close my eyes and know where her hands are even when she is not touching me! She has helped me with visualization and increasing energy in my body. I find the work directed specifically at my abdomen to be the most helpful.

My head had been feeling very foggy, heavy, and unclear. I had also a slight headache. I told her this and she worked on my head and shoulders. We worked to unblock my circulation in my neck and shoulders and worked at taking out all toxins from my head and sending in new energy. The difference after the session was amazing! My head felt clear for the first time in days and stayed clear.

> *This treatment with Erin was four days post chemo. She told me that her head felt "heavy" so a simple brain balancing and mind clearing did wonders to rid her of the internal chatter and open space for new clarity. Erin was very receptive and I thoroughly enjoyed our session.*

March 10, 1998

Wow! I'm really stressed out tonight. It's very difficult to deal with the fact that so many people are all of a sudden making decisions in my life. I understand now how hard this is going to be over the next several months – everyone trying to help in their own way puts a new demand on me.

There are so many appointments, people to call, people to explain everything to, people concerned, allow for this and allow for that. There are more and more factors to take into consideration. AAARRRGGG!!! Okay, take a deep breath – pull back all my energy. My energy is mine, I need to keep it. I know everyone is just trying to help but they're sucking away all my energy! It's mine – you can't have it. I will meditate before going to sleep tonight to re-energize.

March 12, 1998

I had a couple of bad dreams last night; I guess it's to be expected after the stress of yesterday. I went to bed and visualized for one hour. I was pretty upset about feeling a loss of control.

March 13, 1998

I can't wear a hat every day and just hope that the wig looks good. I know that hair loss is all part of this but I'm afraid of looking really sick. I look good and feel good – hopefully that won't change. I feel really good! I actually forget that I have this horrible disease sometimes. I know and expect this to get a lot harder than it is right now but I am strong and will win. I am willing to fight for my life – no holds barred.

March 15, 1998

This last visit with Alma was quite amazing. She put her hands on my stomach and we worked on directing energy into my stomach, to take out any toxins and put in good energy to raise the vibration which cancer cells don't like! My stomach actually got hot! I could physically feel the energy inside my stomach – it was amazing! I left feeling more energized and a little more at peace. I find the sessions are very calming.

> *Treatment day with Erin was always filled with the unexpected. Today she was on her way to work and arrived full of chatter and lightness. She looked striking in her business attire, sporting her new wig and hat, and nonchalantly flung them both on the couch as she climbed onto the therapy table. This easy going, curious persona was always delightful to work with.*

CHAPTER 2

Discovering Purpose

"I get up, I walk, I fall down, meanwhile I keep dancing"

March 19, 1998

It's the funniest thing! I am fighting the fight of my life – it's mentally exhausting, but I'm sooo happy! I know I'm changed forever, I know my family and friends are changed forever, but I'm having so much fun with life. I wake up every day and thank God for another day and the strength to get through it. He has been there for me every day, helping me to cope with this journey.

I am awed by my body, its healing and its strength. It truly is a temple, a piece of perfection we all have a tendency to take advantage of.

The happiness is deep, honest, and true. I am thoroughly enjoying the craziness of work. I am awed by my body, its healing and its strength. It truly is a temple, a piece of perfection we all have a tendency to take advantage of. I have a new-found respect for the complexities of the human body. Its creation really is an absolute masterpiece.

I'm really enjoying my friends. All of them, and of course my beautiful sister, are my Circle of Love. I am so lucky. You know that saying "If you don't have your health, you don't have anything" – It's not true!

Unfortunately or fortunately, it's when you don't have your health that you discover and truly appreciate things in your life you may have taken for granted. My social calendar is very full even now and will stay that way.

LIFE, DESPITE EVERYTHING, IS TRULY GOOD RIGHT NOW!

Now for a tiny bit of negative chatter. I haven't been sleeping for two nights now. I have been having very bad dreams. I don't know exactly why. My dreams always seem to begin with me running for my life. I'm running from what appears to be an unseen danger. There are a lot of people in my dreams who I do not recognize.

March 20, 1998

I am very tired and with my tiredness comes shortness and impatience. I had blood tests and a meeting with Dr. H. today. Mom and Dad were both with me. My blood tests showed that my white cell count (immune system) is down so my chemo has been postponed for a week. I will have chemo every 4 weeks now. My cancer markers have fallen from 80 to 50. So the bottom line is that all is working the way it should.

This is the happiest and saddest time of my life!

When I'm tired I don't want anyone around. That I find, happens a lot now. If I am tired, I need to be alone – no phones, no people. I can't handle any type of noise or voices or proximity to someone. I need silence and aloneness. I feel badly about that. I know I get uptight and even rude but it is just there.

This is the happiest and saddest time of my life!

March 22, 1998

I woke up still feeling very sad. I cried a little bit more and found myself looking through my album at all the cards that everyone has sent me over these weeks. It is absolutely overwhelming to me, the support that I am getting. I can't believe how many people, even those I do not know, are thinking and praying for me. I received a card from my aunt's friend, whom I've never met, offering support and some meditation ideas. It's amazing. I can feel the support and positive energy coming my way from across the country. It really does make a difference. The positive vibes and karma, if you will, can be felt from everywhere. I feel blessed at this awful time in my life, to be so loved. This is the best of times and worst of times all at once. I am forever changed by this experience. It just may be the best thing that ever happened to me.

I can feel the support and positive energy coming my way from across the country. It really does make a difference. The positive vibes and karma, if you will, can be felt from everywhere. I feel blessed at this awful time in my life, to be so loved.

March 25, 1998

Alma was amazing as usual. She opened up my middle chakras so that we could focus on filling my body full of new energy. When she used her crystal at the beginning of the session, my energy was completely shut down. We worked on filling me up. She also worked on my pancreas and spleen to release all the toxins. This felt very good today. When she did the initial dragging off of the toxins across my whole body, I could feel the pulling happening inside. It was an amazing feeling. Actually, what I noticed today is that whenever she would clean an area, the area and my skin would feel cool. It was a very distinct feeling. One minute my body was warm and as she dragged off the toxins, it cooled. Awesome!

The "toxins" that Erin refers to are from the chemo which is poisonous to the whole body. I worked at pulling them from the immune system so it wasn't weakened any further then energized the chemo to give it more power in the area of the cancer.

March 29, 1998

I SHAVED MY HEAD!! My hair had started to thin rather quickly around March 20th. I got really tired of picking hair off myself, all day, it was everywhere around the apartment. It still looked okay but it was turning into a real pain so I told my sister to cut it off. It was hilarious! We both were laughing sooo hard! I put a towel around my shoulders and sat in my kitchen on a stool. I gave her my scissors and she went to town! She cut off all my hair as close to the scalp as possible. It was very important to me to maintain as much control over every part of my life and this disease. I cut my hair short before I had to. I shaved my head before I had to. I believe that action is very important. This way I do things my own way, in my own time, and then the disease is not dictating my life experiences to me. My head feels better now. I would recommend that anyone who is going to lose their hair take things into their own hands and shave it before it falls out.

March 30, 1998

I find myself appreciating life each moment so much more than ever. This is a very odd thing. The ups and downs are exhausting. When I'm up I'm actually almost giggly. I find myself thinking and remembering times and situations and just laughing out loud about them when no one else is around. I don't have a lot of down times. The hardest times are when I'm tired. As with anyone, I'm more vulnerable when I'm tired and that's when I cry or feel depressed. But it really doesn't happen often.

I find myself appreciating life each moment so much more than ever. This is a very odd thing.

My moods are generally quite good. I think my friends have a lot to do with it! It is great when everyone around you is in awe of you and your attitude. I feel incredibly undeserving of this because I think that anyone would do what they had to, to get by. But I know that some people are always very negative and down when they go through this. I think those people are sunk before they even start. I'm having quite an incredible experience with this and intend to keep treating it that way all the way through. I am learning so much about myself and my Inner Self.

This is a very lonely journey in some ways. There are so many people with so much love all around me and yet most of my strength and attitude has to come from me. This disease has transformed me into much more of an introverted person than I ever was. I think you have to be alone because the chemo makes you very irritable and short tempered on some days. You have to really know yourself and be honest with others about your moods.

This is a very lonely journey in some ways. There are so many people with so much love all around me and yet most of my strength and attitude has to come from me.

April 5, 1998

I'm feeling quite guilty that I haven't written in my journal for so long, I just haven't been feeling like I want to.

My second round of chemo was postponed for a week because my blood counts were too low. I was a little disappointed to learn that my subsequent treatments would now come every four weeks instead of every three but it's nice to have the extra week – makes life seem a little more normal. It allows me to work a lot, which is good and bad.

I'm having a really hard time drawing the line between work hours and social life. I know I'm not spending enough time alone like this doing things just for me! I don't know why I remain so incredibly active. I think it is a way of maintaining normality in my life. Also, I feel that this is my life and I don't want to put it on hold for this disease. I'm doing almost as much as I did before this all happened – much to everyone's dismay. I keep being told by everyone to relax and slow down but I just don't want to! I do when I feel really tired. I try to listen to my body and rest when needed. I do sleep a lot I find – at least ten hours per night. I do my prayers and some visualization every night and sometimes in the morning but I know I should do more. There is just no time!!

April 6, 1998

The nausea in the second round of chemo was quite a bit worse than the first round. It was manageable initially but by the end of the week and throughout the weekend it was worse. I find the second week after a chemo week, the one where my blood work and immune system go way down, is very difficult. The week right after chemo is high energy, and then I fall, along with my blood work. This past one was very difficult. My attention span dropped considerably. I could not focus on work for more than four to five hours. My patience was very low and I cried quite a bit. It was a very emotional week. It's funny, because I wasn't feeling sorry for myself when I cried. Many times I don't even know why I cried. I think I spent most of the week being tired. I start to feel frustrated that I just can't keep up to everything I want to do and I feel just tired of all of this – tired of living in this body. It's often difficult to explain. It's just a feeling of loss, of despair.

April 7, 1998

I had my first group session with Alma and three other therapists. It was amazing. I had four women doing Healing Touch at once. I was re-energized fully! The sensations were incredible – so much energy from their hands. When they worked at releasing all the toxins from areas, the areas would turn cold as they finished. It was an amazing feeling. They cleared my head of fogginess, released all toxins that I didn't need and I actually felt lighter as the session went on.

This sensation is one of the most powerful feelings I always come away with from Healing Touch sessions. I go in feeling 'heavy' is the best way to describe it and when I leave I feel lighter. When they rake their hands over my energy field to cleanse me of unwanted and unneeded toxins I actually can feel the weight being taken off my body. They said in that particular session that there was a lot of emotional energy being cleansed. I believe that is the main reason for my being so emotional at certain times. The Healing Touch brings a lot of emotional energy that is blocked and stored in my abdominal area, to the surface. So usually about 1-2 days after Healing Touch I am quite weepy. I'm grateful to them for helping me to release all these feelings because I think that blocked emotions are a part of what can cause disease.

Alma and the group did a lot of work on my left side during this visit as well. Ultrasound and chest x-rays all came back normal and Dr. H. couldn't tell me why my side was so sore. The therapists used a very powerful crystal on my side and told me a lot of cleansing was being done.

April 9, 1998

I was very busy the next week getting ready for Monk's anniversary party. I was beginning to feel better this week, stronger and not so nauseous. It was a great success! I had dinner with several friends before the party then at 9 pm it began! What fun! I can't believe it lasted so long. I danced until 2 am! I think it had a lot to do with the Healing Touch treatment I had that afternoon, the way you would go to get a massage to relax and rejuvenated – well I go to Healing Touch.

This one was particularly interesting because they found a "spike" in my energy field on my left side where all the pain had been. This appointment was an incredible experience! I closed my eyes and could feel when this one therapist moved her hand around the spike. When her hand went one way, the pain went the same way. When she moved another way, the pain traveled with her hand. My eyes were closed!! And yet I could tell where her hand was. And my spike was 4 feet off my body – that is where her hand was! We worked a lot on that area that day. She says a spike is a hole in your energy field. It could have been caused by an accident that had physical consequences or may have been emotional trauma (if the spike is in the emotional centre). She repaired the spike as best as could be.

The next group session was with two therapists. The spike was still there but was a little better than the previous appointment. It's actually not hurting at all right now so who knows what really makes it better.

April 24, 1998

I'm still brought to tears by the incredible amount of support I have from all around. Dad mentioned that he had run into several people in the last couple of days, people who don't know me but know of me through Dad. One of the couples said that every morning, they get down on their knees and pray for me! I don't even know these people! Another couple that lives down the lane from him said they think about me every day and hope I am okay.

I appreciate every moment and am very conscious of not doing anything or saying anything that would make me want to take that moment back.

I just can't get used to these things. I well up inside just thinking about it. I'm having a hard time just keeping up with the phone messages from well wishers and sending thank you cards for the gifts.

I really notice the change physically and emotionally. Life is different now. I'm actually literally stopping to smell the flowers as I walk. I love being outside and breathing deeply. I appreciate every moment and am very conscious of not doing anything or saying anything that would make me want to take that moment back. I'm working a lot and loving it although I do wish I could work more. Right now I work five days a week, usually six to seven hours a day, with the odd twelve-hour-day. I don't work the week of chemo. I feel like I want to work more but my body just gets so tired. It really comes on all of a sudden. It's like hitting a physical wall. One minute I'm okay and then the next I have to leave RIGHT NOW!!

I love my body – it is my temple and must be treated that way. My body is fighting a very strong fight – a good fight – and for that I love it very much

I'm becoming very pensive – I think a lot about life and about my friends. Songs have taken on new meanings for me.

When I hear Sarah McLaughlin's song, "I will remember you – will you remember me?" I think how I would like it played at my funeral – yet I don't think about dying. Anything but coming through this ordeal healthy is not an option. I feel I must teach others how to be strong through this. I say to myself "I have cancer" and it sounds so foreign! It's not that I don't believe it or that I'm in denial, it's just that it sounds surreal. I'm so active professionally and socially that I feel like I'm just being side-tracked for awhile – nothing major! We'll see what I think in a few months!

It is my journey, though I did not choose it, I welcome it and all the hardship it presents. It is my faith and my soul.

Another song of Sarah's that gets to me on my bad days is, "I'm just tired of living in here" referring to her own body. That's how I feel sometimes, when I feel like my body is letting me down but then I rethink that. I love my body – it is my temple and must be treated that way. My body is fighting a very strong fight – a good fight – and for that I love it very much.

I was at the Cancer Clinic on Friday and the doctor told me my cancer markers were down into a normal range and everything looked good. All news was very good, very positive. At one point during the exam she remarked that there are things that I can do to make my scar fade or not be as noticeable. I jumped right in. As far as I'm concerned, I will NEVER do a thing to minimize that scar. I LOVE MY SCAR. It represents everything I am going through. When this is over, it will be a reminder of the fight of my life, my incredible journey and all that was involved. Every inch of that scar is symbolic of life, a life almost lost, a fight for health, purity, happiness, endurance, and a representation of strength in me that I never knew existed.

It is my journey, though I did not choose it, I welcome it and all the hardship it presents. It is my faith and my soul.

April 25, 2004

I'm mad at everyone today – since last night actually, I desperately wish for 'normal' in my life and without hair it doesn't seem possible. I just spent a wonderful afternoon with friends. After such a great day why do I feel so angry? I wish I had a kick bag here right now because I would really work it! I laughed so hard all day – really laughed – and now I'm just angry. I feel lonely and alone in this. I feel an incredible need to go away – just take off from all of this shit. I feel very self-conscious, like I'm never totally relaxed. My hairlessness is always on my mind and no matter how much everyone says it looks great and I look great and blah, blah, blah – what the fuck else are they going to say? That I don't look good?

I feel trapped. I think that's what it is. I am here watching everyone's life move along, progress, change, and I am stuck in a Cancer Hell.

I feel trapped. I think that's what it is. I am here watching everyone's life move along, progress, change, and I am stuck in a Cancer Hell – getting less attractive, feeling less attractive, and knowing that there is no prospect of love for a very long time. After all, who would want a bald, sick woman in their life? My friend's careers are progressing, and I'm just trying to hold onto mine. They are getting more and more physically fit – I'm just trying to get enough sleep at night. I feel lost. I want desperately to run away, to a cottage style house in the country, with two labs, maybe a horse, and just retreat within myself.

Wow! I'm feeling really sorry for myself tonight. I could start listing all the things in my life that I am thankful for – which would fill the rest of this book – but then there's the CANCER that overshadows all of the rest.

It's just not something that you can get past. I know that when this is over, even now to a certain degree, I will almost be thankful that it happened. But right now it's bad, very bad.

And I know it's something that I will have to live with for the rest of my life, counting the days, months, hopefully years, of remission, just waiting for it to recur and take my life. I MISS MY BABIES…….

April 26, 1998

I was a little stressed about Dad coming over today, for the night. I know he really wants to stay involved but I find I need a lot of time alone. I was cranky when I spoke to him on the phone today so he immediately called Lara and expressed his concerns that I may not be okay. I don't know how to make him understand that my moods change almost hourly. I can be happy, sad, angry, jealous and depressed all in the same morning. It's all par-for-the-course in my life right now. Dad getting stressed about it only makes me stressed. I'll have to try to explain things to him better.

May 10, 1998

You know, I find it really hard to remember how sick I am when I'm having this much fun! Everyone around me is amazed at how much energy I have because I go, go, go all the time. Some of my healthy friends can't keep up with me. I just got back from Seattle from an overnight 'restaurant tour and shop-till-you-drop expedition.' We had a lot of fun! Last week work was busy and I was in every day.

May 11, 1998

I'm not afraid of dying – I'm afraid of the process of dying. I just watched the movie One Night Stand, and it has put me in a very weird space. It preaches life is short, get your shit straightened out and figured out. I'm very tired this week.

I know my blood counts are low, I can feel it physically and emotionally. It puts me in a bad place – very alone, very pensive. Nothing matters to me.

Sometimes I just don't know why this is happening to me – am I going to die from this? Is that really what is in store for this soul, this life on earth – could it be that all is for naught? Are our lives predestined, predetermined? I don't think that I believe that. I can't allow myself to think that because then there would be no point in fighting this evil. I'm just really tired and that seems to make me philosophical about all that is happening to me.

May 12, 1998

Alma pulled a lot of crap from my liver today! She said it felt prickly and thick. That could also be what is making me feel so emotional. I felt a lot of pulling around my liver and spleen while she worked today. She was away all last week. Even though I had a lot of energy last week it was a 'heavy' sort of energy. I miss the raking and pulling away of the toxins when I don't see her for awhile. It really makes a difference – she takes away the heaviness that I feel from chemo. When she worked on my liver today she said she could smell something coming from me. It seems it was the toxins that were being released from my liver.

May 14, 1998

I had to cancel plans for tomorrow night with friends because I'm afraid I won't be up for it. It really depresses me. This round of chemo is definitely harder than the last round and I'm afraid of what's to come. The really tough stuff, Taxol, hasn't started yet and I'm afraid of it.

One minute I know I can do this and the next minute I'm afraid that I can't. God, please help me. I'm so jealous of my friends – it's getting harder and harder to be around them. I'm very sad.

May 15, 1998

I woke up feeling considerably better today. It seems that when the energy comes back, it comes back with a vengeance! I worked all day today, came home for two hours and went back tonight for a few hours. I actually forget what I'm going through, just for a while, and then it creeps back. I'm scared of what is to come. I'm excited at what is to come. All are possibilities. There are no guarantees one way or the other. I never in my life thought I would find myself in this place. What a strange place to be. I do enjoy this level of consciousness and spirituality I have reached. It is generally so positive. Everything is so important now!

I do enjoy this level of consciousness and spirituality I have reached. It is generally so positive. Everything is so important now!

May 16 to 25, 1998

I met an old boyfriend today and the feeling of romance returned with abundance. We went home together, had a long talk about the relationship we don't have and ended up in bed together –

again. This night was the first time I have had sex since the operation and to my relief everything still works the way it used to! No problems with anything! I don't think I would have wanted it to happen with anyone else. He was so gentle and understanding that I began to feel like a whole person again. It was a beautiful experience and one I needed so badly. I thought I would have a lot of inhibitions about hair loss, the scar etcetera but I didn't.

Well, another uplifting discussion with Dr. H. I always feel so hopeless when I talk to him. He basically told me that because the chemo to date has not shrunk the remaining tumour that it probably has not had much effect on the other stuff in my abdominal wall. He was so negative that I felt like I had been hit with a bat. He said that if it turns out I would need a colostomy – not to have the surgery because it would not increase my chances much anyway. I was devastated! Absolutely devastated!

No matter how many people are around to help me fight this, it's ultimately a very lonely battle. At the beginning and end of each day, it's just me, mind, body and soul, trying desperately to accept and make sense of this.

The rest of the week was a blur. Dr. H. left me feeling hopeless, depressed, and stuck. I spent the week working on my attitude and little else. I can't believe the change in my mindset that that appointment caused. Maybe now that I have a better perspective, I think that it may have been God's way of making me take all of this more seriously.

June 1, 1998

I will not be spending much of my time at work anymore. I can't justify spending energy on anything other than me and my health. Everything I do now is related to that. I have and will not allow any stresses in my life, including work.

I honestly never expected this day to come – the day when I would choose to leave my job. This is what Dr. H. said when he said you just can't concentrate on it. It's not the drugs, or treatment or program I am on – it's priorities. Everything takes a back seat to my life right now. I am extremely self-involved where everything I do is about me maintaining a positive attitude and beating this horrendous disease. Nothing else matters. The fear alone is paralyzing.

I'm just not ready to die yet. I honestly think that I am open to feeling it but I don't. I feel like I still have a lot to do in this life and this just isn't my time. I hope and pray my body allows me to fulfill my life's purpose. I will do whatever I have to help it heal and regenerate itself.

I believe from all the reading I have been doing and my gut instinct, that I must accompany the surgeries and chemo with a nutritional plan, a very strict one, administered by a doctor to help my body's own natural healing powers. I will continue the Healing Touch also. I hope that the combination of all of these will be enough along with my own visualization to fight this disease. God, please help me.

No matter how many people are around to help me fight this, it's ultimately a very lonely battle. At the beginning and end of each day, it's just me, mind, body and soul, trying desperately to accept and make sense of this.

June 14, 1998

I have spent morning to night researching various alternative nutritional treatments available. The more I read about them the more I want to believe in them. I have consulted with a couple of nutritionists that have the audacity to say that they don't even consider cancer to be a serious disease anymore because they have healed it so many times. How can I ignore this information? I know the conventional doctors will not even give this the time of day. My whole family met last weekend to go over the information and all were in favour of the Metabolic Program.

It is chemistry-based and uses a multitude of vitamins and minerals several times a day accompanied by cleansing enemas. The purpose is to completely detoxify the body then build it back up with the vitamins and minerals needed to bring the body to a healthy state for fighting disease.

The Cancer Agency had a conference with all the top radiologists and surgeons to discuss my case.

Their unanimous decision was for further surgery to remove the remaining tumour and to continue with chemo. My Dad asked them if there was anything I could be doing with respect to my diet and nutrition to help things along and their response was no! I could not believe it! There is incontrovertible evidence showing that cancer is caused by a deficient immune system. This system is built up by excellent nutrition and diet – they directly affect it. So how can they dismiss this so easily? Is it my destiny to fight for alternative medicine? They just don't see it.

This is a very lonely battle. It is the hardest decision I have ever had to make. Do I go with nutrition, surgery and/or chemo? It's so hard to walk away from conventional medicine when it has been ingrained in your head all your life that when you have cancer, you get chemo – end of story.

Erin wove her way through the value of alternative versus conventional medicine and its challenging decisions. Healing Touch did not require her to make an either / or decision about her treatments but the nutritional program did. Erin decided to hold off on further surgery and chemo until she had time to fully experience the benefits of the nutritional / metabolic program. This was a very difficult decision for her. What she hoped for was a meeting-of-the-minds toward the nutritional program and conventional medicine.

CHAPTER 3

Looking for Options

"What you feel in emotions is the answer – you have to remember what the question is."

June 17, 1998

Big day! I signed on to start metabolic therapy. Dr. F. says he can cure cancer – so we'll see! I am going into this with my whole heart and soul. I really feel good about having made the decision to use alternative medicine and to have chosen this particular therapy. I believe in what I am doing. I am postponing surgery and chemo indefinitely right now and I am going to see what the next 12 weeks brings.

I had a very cool visualization experience two days ago that really confirmed for me that trying something alternative right now is the right thing to do. It goes like this: I took myself out of my body and made myself tiny so that I could go back inside my body to look around at everything. I entered through my ear, went down my throat, looked at my clear lungs, clear liver and spleen. I then went to the site of the remaining tumour. I looked around it. It looked grey with an unsmooth surface. It is oblong in shape. I stood there, along my bowels, looking at the tumour and asked my body what it wants me to do in order to get rid of this cancer. The thing that came into my mind was "I WANT A SALAD."

Salads have always represented health food to me and I intuitively knew that my body was asking me to feed it a metabolic program with strict diet and supplements to really pump it up.

That visualization exercise was pivotal to me. I knew that my body was asking a for a less toxic, healthy alternative to chemo. I have decided to honour that request.

June 18, 1998

My healing appointments have been wonderful. I know that Healing Touch has helped me to keep feeling so good throughout all of this. Alma has kept my liver and spleen clear by pulling away all the toxins of the chemo. The lymphatic drains and the raking have pulled away a lot of chemical and emotional CRAP. From this work I have learned how to be in touch with my body, to really listen to it and to trust my intuitive side. This last one is and has been fundamental to my progress mentally. Your body and subconscious mind, which could also be your intuitive side, are very powerful. I am so grateful for this lesson. I do trust myself and I try to do what my body tells me to do.

From this work I have learned how to be in touch with my body, to really listen to it and to trust my intuitive side. This last one is and has been fundamental to my progress mentally.

I now also understand that when my liver is sore it may not be from filtering chemo but filtering stress and emotional crap that overloads it. We are always too quick to assume that our aches and pains are related to something we ate, or in my case, the work my body has to do to get through the chemo. In actuality, my liver and spleen have been sore lately because I have spent the last three weeks doing incredible amounts of reading, research and soul searching to decide the course of my treatment.

This has been emotionally exhausting and extremely stressful. Alma pointed out today that the liver filters everything INCLUDING emotions. I couldn't understand why my liver would be sore today because chemo had been over for almost three weeks. So it makes sense that it's the emotional things that are hard on my liver right now.

June 21, 1998

I called Dad to say Happy Father's Day and my nice positive little world came tumbling down! Once again we were back to untrusting, suspicious, negativity about the new program. He wants to know how many people have been sick on this program and could we get Dr. F. to sign a contract saying that if I get sick we get our money back. I cried all the way home from my sister's. I have to have a serious talk with Dad tonight and explain how much I need his support. I cannot have someone in my life right now that can inflict such stress on me, even though he doesn't mean to. The rest of the day with friends helped my attitude and there was a message of apology from Dad when I got home.

June 25, 1998

Well, I've been doing the metabolic therapy for four days. The first two days were okay but Wednesday was awful! I felt bloated and had a headache all day. It was all I could do to take all the pills and not throw up! It is quite an incredible process. I actually feel like I have more energy when I'm not feeling well. It is a real mind-over-matter situation. It is definitely going to be a tough summer but I have no doubt in my mind that this will work.

June 28, 1998

People are funny – you really find out who you can count on at times like these. People have this idea that 'being there' for someone with an illness means saying "Call me if you need anything." Or making a token phone call every other day. This past weekend for example no one came by to visit. To me, everyone knows I can't really go anywhere. I have bits and pieces of this program that must be done practically every hour. So 'being there' for me, is not inviting me out to a beer garden, but coming to see me.

I am learning some painful lessons that will forever change my life and my perspective on 'being there' for others. I want to share this new found insight with others in my position. I want to use this knowledge to work with others in crisis.

I am learning some painful lessons that will forever change my life and my perspective on 'being there' for others. I want to share this new found insight with others in my position. I want to use this knowledge to work with others in crisis. I must survive in order to accomplish what I know and believe, is my true purpose in life. To do the work that God intended me to do. I truly appreciate and love all that I am learning – even though it can be bittersweet at times.

June 29, 1998

No matter how much research I've done on soul searching, doubt has a way of worming its way into my mind every now and then. I don't doubt my decision to go with metabolic therapy but I think my concern is my own body. I know my body, on its own, can turn this around. I just wonder if it can in time.

I feel a little nervous right now because my insides hurt. My colon, intestine, liver, pancreas and spleen are all working very hard with a lot of new materials.

They are complaining a fair amount. I just hope all this is okay and that I am not doing any harm to myself. I think if I didn't have this last tumour I wouldn't be so nervous. I am obsessed with eliminating all toxins from my body. I guess that's a good thing but I think its also what makes me nervous – when I'm afraid its not working to the best of my ability.

I'm also worried about my relationships. I find everything so superficial. I was upset this weekend about not being invited out on Saturday but today when I found out what they did I was glad I wasn't there! It's the same old bar scene: too many cocktails and drooling over some guy. I am really afraid I'm going to progress along this path that I'm on and end up having no interest in my friends anymore. I recently realized what a totally superficial life I lived, they still do, and I have no interest in returning to it. I really enjoy my own company.

I'm tired now – See you tomorrow E xoxo (that's for my body, because it rocks!!)

July 1, 1998

Wow – I have so many feelings about so many things. I feel like I don't have sure footing on any front now. Right now I desperately wish I had tried a different kind of life. I feel in my gut that I belong in the country, with fields and forests and mountains right outside my front door to go walking in forever. I really need that right now. I feel like I no longer belong where I am, in this life I loved so much. A part of me actually feels like if I had my way, my place in the country or mountains and a wholesome life, that I would have a better chance of beating this.

I seem to be losing all interest in anything a city has to offer. It's all so superficial. It would be a quiet kind of life, but this present life is getting lonely! I can't relate to anyone anymore. I know I have all the answers inside me; I'm having trouble reaching them right now. I can't hear myself very well right now. It's not about finding a cure for this disease anymore; it's about living day to day.

I don't know what my place is in this world anymore. Maybe that's the point. Maybe I no longer have a place in this world. Maybe this is what happens when it's just time to go? Although, deep down, I really don't feel that and I don't think I believe it either. I see myself so clearly living a completely different life and I do feel like I still have so much to offer people with life-threatening illnesses. My problem is I have no reference of time. I can't seem to see when this is going to happen. I am getting a stronger and stronger feeling that I don't belong in the life I am in, or was living, any more. Circumstances have to change.

As serious as this disease is, I don't feel that I can put my life on hold while I try to beat it! It seems to me that the transformation to a new life is a large part of the cure. The problem is I don't know where to go.

I see myself so clearly living a completely different life and I do feel like I still have so much to offer people with life-threatening illnesses.

It's amazing how defined we all are by what we do and where we go and who our friends are. Once that's all gone and it's just you and yourself in this private little world, you really begin to look at yourself as a person and think about what you really want out of life. All that other stuff just takes your mind off of what your purpose in life should be.

It's good at keeping your mind occupied so that any introspection that is done is fairly superficial and very limited at that. That is how I lived all through my twenties 'til now – very busy, popular, great times, great friends, took what I wanted when I wanted it.

I never really and truly dealt with issues in my life like my parents divorce; sibling problems; relationship problems; marrying for the wrong reasons and allowing my husband to control my life, my thoughts, my dreams and my goals. All of these events in my life and the fact that I did not deal with them properly, I believe, are part of the reason for my current illness. What a tremendous amount of shit to go through in eight or nine short years. Yes I believe that the Powers That Be have kicked me in the head to say "Get your shit together and fix your life!!!" With this said, how could I ever go back to my life as it was before this happened? I cannot.

Be true to yourself! I don't think I have ever really done that except for the day I left my husband. That may have been the most honest day of my life to date (excluding the last five months).

July 2, 1998

This metabolic program is so hard and I am so determined to get through it though. I thoroughly believe in it. I just wish my bowels were functioning properly.

I read the animal cards last night in search for an answer of whether I am doing the right thing. It basically signifies TRUST & SURRENDER yourself to the future, what the Universe has in mind for you. That keeps coming up everywhere, intuitively and through the cards.

July 6, 1998

I got very upset and stressed after speaking to Dad today because he wanted to sit down with Mom and me to totally discuss my finances and budget.

I guess he has a right to know this given that he helps to support me but I felt so invaded and violated. I have endured five-and-a-half months of being poked, prodded, examined, and discussed as well as having my bowel movements as a topic of conversation with everyone. I just want something ANYTHING to be mine! I want some part of my life, ANY PART, to be just mine and nobody else's business!

Once again, Alma helped me to see that I do have something that is just mine; I have my thoughts, my soul and my feelings.

Once again, Alma helped me to see that I do have something that is just mine; I have my thoughts, my soul and my feelings. Those I can have and no one can share them unless I decide to let them! That does make me feel a little better – Alma is good at that.

Then Dad also said that he worries that I'm not eating right! I almost flipped! What the fuck does he think I'm doing? I know that it's just him being his usual control freak but I might have to have another chat with him. The last thing I need is anyone not believing that I can handle this program! Well I'll show him and everyone!

You don't scare me!!

July 7, 1998

Alma and I are working on releasing old stresses. Every cell in your body has memory and they hold in the memories of your entire life and past lives! So as I rebuild my body with the nutritional program I want to rebuild my emotional self at a cellular level as well. This entails releasing all old stresses, frustrations and negative feelings. Most of these surround my abdominal or emotional chakra.

July 9, 1998

I feel like I've had an emotional breakthrough today. I saw Dr. B. yesterday and she confirmed that the tumour was no better and no worse than my previous exam. She also confirmed that there was no blockage in my bowel. Before seeing her I had convinced myself that my bowel movement problems were caused by the tumour having grown. I think I actually caused my constipation by mentally believing that there was a blockage.

Today I had two bowel movements. It renewed my faith in what I am doing and convinced me that the constipation was diet-related and not tumour-related. I hope I can maintain this mental attitude. I got lost for a while there, in the last few days.

I think working with Alma this week has also really helped. We've been working on my abdominal area to release any pent-up aggressions or negative feelings that I may have stored up in there. We went right back to when I was three years old. She said she felt me releasing negative energy all the way through. I've had a great life so far, in general but a very emotionally-charged one that I haven't always dealt with very well. I am going to work on this.

The beautiful thing about releasing old stuff is that you don't have to be specific or re-live the bad times in your life. You can just focus on 'letting go' of all negative stress that is tied up in your cells, organs, body and field. I think I have a lot of shit inside but I know I'm getting better. I see these next months as a total body cleansing, body and soul.

> *It was a joy to watch Erin integrate the energy work into her life. Like a sponge, she absorbed every detail then practiced it and shared it. She was becoming a powerful teacher*

I had great social energy today chatting with several friends and playing telephone tag with others.

All in all a great day! I'm still not ready to resume any kind of active social life though. It's just too hard with all this nutritional stuff happening as well.

July 13, 1998

I feel quite alone in this – it's a weird type of alone though. I am not running to find a support group. I quite enjoy being by myself. I'm okay with it. I have the odd social day when I speak to and socialize with people just to keep in touch but for the most part, I just keep to myself. I feel bad about myself sometimes because my eczema is really bad.

Apparently it's all part of the detox but I have a fear that it will never go away and that I will come out of all this scarred on my skin forever. For some reason that scares me more than the cancer. I guess it's just another lesson to learn. I am more than how I look physically and I know that, but I would really like to keep looking good, which in turn helps me feel good – or is it vice versa?

I guess it's just another lesson to learn. I am more than how I look physically and I know that, but I would really like to keep looking good, which in turn helps me feel good – or is it vice versa?

July 14, 1998

Turning Point ***** I was lying in bed doing some visualization and prayer asking and seeking for the cancer to disappear. All of a sudden a strong feeling of a wave passed right over and through me. I saw myself very clearly being back at work, enjoying my job and living very healthy and happy. I also saw no cancer where the cancer had been. As of that moment, my cancer was gone. There was only blackness where the remaining tumour used to be. I saw myself anew – very healthy, never to be sick again. I had a very cleansed emotional, spiritual, intellectual and physical body. It was the first time that I actually saw a light at the end of the tunnel. I saw my life after cancer. I could never see that before!

The feeling is overwhelming! It is so strong and so full of happiness. As of today I consider the cancer gone and feel and see a whole new perspective to this journey I am on. It's all about the metabolic program – rebuilding a sick body to the peak of health. I feel I am on the verge of major discoveries and moments. I know that as of right now my whole life and perspective has changed. My intuition and my body are telling me that the cancer is gone.

July 15, 1998

I just had the most incredible session with Alma! I had a feeling last night as I lay awake, that I was on the verge of major discoveries. Well was I right! This is the most incredible day I have had since all this began. I don't know where to begin, I'm so excited.

I guess the beginning is to say that I have felt for a few days now that a major part of my recovery has to be a total emotional baggage cleansing. So Alma and I have been working on releasing stuff into her hands, usually from my abdominal area (which is your emotional centre) and it's been going well. I've been practicing at home as well. My body has been feeling very busy energetically since I started the metabolic program – very different from when I was on chemo. At that time I just felt shut down.

Anyway, today when Alma asked what I wanted to work on I said I wanted to do more releasing. She felt that, at this point in my illness and subsequent healing, that I was now ready to delve into more specific emotional trauma areas and work on dealing with and releasing the pent up feelings associated with it. We began working on my frustrations with Mom and Dad right now and I learned what she calls 'mirroring'.

She explained that when someone is really making you angry or is frustrating you, it is usually because something in their behaviour or what they are saying is common to your own personality, or is a truth you have to learn about yourself. So what I have to do to deal with those frustrations is when it is happening, is to turn around, look at myself and ask what is it about what he/she is saying that is true to my own personality. This helps me to understand why it frustrates me or makes me angry and helps me deal with my own feelings.

Next came the big stuff. It wasn't as much what she said but what it all makes me realize. That is one of the beautiful things about Alma. She has a comforting soothing voice and a way of asking gentle questions that really put you on the right track. She can pull things out of me without my even realizing what has happened.

She explained that when someone is really making you angry or is frustrating you, it is usually because something in their behaviour or what they are saying is common to your own personality, or is a truth you have to learn about yourself.

I think it's mostly because she has taught me how to think and respond intuitively without second guessing. She has taught me how to listen to my Guides and my Angels and to have confidence in what my body is telling me. All the answers lie within me. I just have to learn how to listen.

Alma proceeded to suggest that she and her peers and many in the alternative medical community believe that when a person gets cancer it is because a part of their body wants to die. She then asked me to think about that. After about thirty seconds I realized and began to feel that all of me wanted to die, in some way because of the last twelve years of my life.

I realized that about one year ago I hit rock bottom. I was drinking a lot, partying a lot, working a lot and basically keeping so busy that I wasn't dealing with anything.

I was a shell of a person walking around, really enjoying my new-found life and freedom after my marriage, but, I guess, never having truly dealt with issues over the last twelve years. I have had many traumas and stayed strong through them all, making sure everyone else was okay – everyone except me. I have to interject here; I just remembered another aspect of this session that was very important.

I had mentioned to Alma that I also wanted to work on my shoulders this day. When she laid her hands on them she said she could feel a great weight on them. When asked what I thought it was, the first image that popped into my mind as a huge sign, made out of blocks, which said CANCER. It looked thick and heavy. She asked me to release it and when I started to she immediately felt a lot of energy coming into her hands. I saw the weight lift and float away from my shoulders and it went up towards the sky.

I realized after my session was over how significant this was in light of the previous night's revelation of the cancer having disappeared from my body.

July 19, 1998

From the past Tuesday night to Saturday morning I was flying high. I was so excited about the last few days I could hardly contain myself. Thursday and Friday nights I went out with friends and by Saturday the first level of detox broke and I was starting to feel sick. I was on an emotional tightrope again. I'm close to the edge all the time.

Trust is so big in this. I have to trust my decisions, trust my body and trust my intuition to tell me if change is required.

Everything I was so excited about last week is still there for me but now I feel frustrated with this program. I know I have to do it and most of me believes that it's the right thing to do but tonight I am scared.

I am scared that the cancer is spreading. I'm scared that it's growing. I keep feeling other symptoms everywhere in my body and don't know if they are real or imagined. I feel like I'm absolutely obsessing.

I am fighting with myself because everything spiritual in me and everything I have asked for intuitively tells me to just TRUST & SURRENDER to the future. Trust is so big in this. I have to trust my decisions, trust my body and trust my intuition to tell me if change is required. I have to trust in my soul and trust in my body to heal itself even though up to now I don't really feel anything happening.

I think that's why its soooo hard. I can't see the change. I think I have seen things in my mind's eye, I believe what I saw, I just don't know if it was what is really happening in my body or what I want and wish to have happening in my body. I have to wait a month for a scan. I must have the answers or I will go nuts in the next month.

July 22, 1998

Trust & Surrender. Trust & Surrender. This is getting really fucking hard. Sometimes I feel like I have one foot nailed to the floor and I'm going around in circles. My bowels have ceased to function properly and that alone distorts everything. This Blind Faith is excruciatingly hard. There's a lot of negativity going on in my brain right now.

I'm trying very hard to, as Alma says, just acknowledge the thoughts and then tell them to leave. I know they do not serve my highest good so I'm not interested in having them in my head right now.

My body never ceases to amaze me. I am truly in awe of it. We are blessed with organs and systems that have intelligence of their own yet work as a team for the whole. We all need to honour and value these attributes early in life.

I'm really sick of the diet. I cheated yesterday and had some cookie dough. I need more willpower. Everyone thinks I am so strong but I'm not always. This program is so hard. It's walking a tightrope and just trusting that angels are there to catch you if you fall, even though you can't see them. It's putting all my faith in God and in my body and I've never done that before.

July 23, 1998

I'm on the ferry to my Dad's in Victoria and feeling tired and nauseous. I believe I'm in the second phase of the detox program. The toxins should be out of my tissues and into my blood. They are now being pushed from my blood into my lymphatic system which will then push them right out of my body. This is the most difficult part for my body and could potentially take the longest. I am almost finished week five out of the twelve programs. It seems to fly by and crawl by all at once.

I think the most difficult aspect of this illness, in true experience from diagnosis till now, is the fact that I have to come to terms with knowing that no matter what I do or how hard I work, it may not be in the cards that I survive this. This is not meant to be negative, it is just the truth that I must accept. It is part of the reason that I try to get the most out of each day.

I tell myself to just look around and enjoy the beautiful day. Be thankful for every moment and every ounce of strength that God has given me – each and every day – to go through this challenge of mine looking great and usually feeling great. It's a lot more than some people can enjoy. My worst days are many people's best days! For this I am eternally grateful.

I am blessed to have been able to maintain a fully functional lifestyle. I am blessed to have the means and support to have been able to quit work to give my full attention to this healing process. There is a song called *Thank You* that I dedicate to everyone in my life. There are so many people, who have helped me through this terrible ordeal. I dedicate it mostly to my own body and God above, both of whom have, so far, been incredible. My body never ceases to amaze me. I am truly in awe of it. We are blessed with organs and systems that have intelligence of their own yet work as a team for the whole. We all need to honour and value these attributes early in life.

I want to make a difference somehow in this regard, this and counseling cancer patients. I must find a way to do both, somehow! This is my goal coming out of this horrendous disease. I think it would be irresponsible of me to do otherwise.

July 24, 1998

When I can't take the pills and the food anymore and I think of skipping a meal, I think of my family; my sister, brother, Mom and Dad and I think of my friends and I have to keep doing it. Through the nausea, headaches and exhaustion I do it anyway. If not for myself, for them.

July 28, 1998

Alma spent two hours on me yesterday doing a lymphatic drain. She has confirmed that the detoxification process has reached my lymphatic system so she pulled toxins out to make room for more energy. I could really feel the heaviness lifting as her work progressed.

I keep thinking, "I want my life back" but it just occurred to me that that is not true. I don't want my old life back – it was unhealthy and untrue. What I really want is my new life to start.

All my chakras were pretty good when we began except for my third one, in my stomach area, which was really erratic. I think it was a fairly heavy detox yesterday and that there was a lot going on in my stomach. By the end of the session it had settled down.

The detox portion of the metabolic program was intense and hard on Erin's lymphatic and digestive system. My heart went out to her as she began to doubt this program. When I held my pendulum over her stomach it went totally chaotic and we just began to laugh. She said it was a true picture of how she felt.

July 29, 1998

Went to Whistler last weekend with The Girls and had a great time. I didn't go to the bar with everyone – it was too hard. Lara stayed in with me and we rented a movie. I had a great time! Lara is awesome in her undying support. I'm bitter and frustrated tonight. I keep thinking, "I want my life back" but it just occurred to me that that is not true. I don't want my old life back – it was unhealthy and untrue. What I really want is my new life to start. I pray every night for the opportunity to start anew and prove to myself and God above and my Angels and my Guides that I can be true to myself, honouring body and soul and have a great, fun, exciting life! I am asking for the opportunity to do it. I am fighting very hard for that time.

I'm fading, must sleep now, Adieu.

July 31, 1998

I hold myself because no one is here to hold me. This is the loneliest battle I could ever imagine. THIS IS SO HARD! I feel like a lost soul fighting for her life in a big, huge world. I feel nondescript, insignificant in the world, yet significant in mine. I cry because I don't think I have done anything so bad in my life to deserve this disease. I have so many prayers, love and friends around me and yet feel deeply and truly alone. I wish someone was here to hug me. This is the worst day yet. My weight is down, my blood pressure is down and eating is very difficult. Self pity has set in.

August 1, 1998

Well I made it through last night but I had to call Lara and Steve to come and stay with me. My blood pressure dropped really low and it kind of scared me. I calmed down once they arrived and I had a fairly good night's sleep. I was pretty sad until they got here.

I totally fucked up today. I had about six cookies and a piece of apple pie. I also skipped my dinner pills. I don't know what's wrong with me. I just rationalized that no matter what happens in the long run today is not going to make or break it. I'm weak. I'm fed up. I feel so out of the loop – whatever the loop is. I failed my 'moment of truth' today. Well, one day at a time and tomorrow is another day.

I've been thinking a lot about starting to write my book.

I went for a walk tonight and ended up down by the water watching the fireworks. It was very lonely. I began crying on the way back, thinking about how sad this disease is. It just never goes away. There is such a thing as getting your mind off it for a while by watching a movie but if there is romance in it at all I can't imagine who is ever going to want to be with me if I can't have kids. I am having a bit of a hard time with feeling like 'damaged goods'.

I am physically and emotionally exhausted. I am hitting some kind of Hopeless Wall. I am so sad. Why me? Why now? Will I survive this? Is this my last summer or my second to last?

There is a huge ball of positive vibes surrounded by the most beautiful strong brilliant white light in me that is buried under shit right now. I know the detox phase is much stronger than previous ones. I think that all these negative, depressing feelings that are coming out of me right now are part of it. I can see that once I get through detox that the brilliant light will shine again.

I have to get these negative feelings out. It's like I have a 'slow leak' with them now. It comes out in waves; usually making me cry for a minute then it subsides. I feel that my sadness at having to go through all this is so overwhelming and so deep and so huge that my mind can only let it out a little at a time or I would just fall apart.

I am not dying. I am living with a degenerating disease – learning how to control it. I want my life back. I demand my life back. I am just thinking that I've never really freaked out about this. Since I went in for surgery – on one level it always seemed surreal, but on a deeper level, very deep, I knew. Before any of this happened I believe my spirit knew. Nothing has ever shocked me, truly, because I knew.

Soulfulness is truly what everything is all about.........

Soulfulness is truly what everything is all about.........

August 2, 1998

I am in hell. Everything is different in this underworld I am in. Colours are different. Feelings are different. Memories are different. There is no rhyme or reason for things. I want desperately to go back to the outer world but I'm not allowed. My conscience won't let me. Let me out!! Let me out!! I'm beginning to question my own strength to go through this and come out a survivor! Anything less is unacceptable – but I don't know how long I can keep fighting.

Life is hell. Life is not hell. Life is beautiful and I thank God for its beauty everyday. This is so drastic, I think I'm manic. My thoughts and feelings change from one second to the next. I'm losing my mind most days.

This round of detox seems to be detoxing my emotional self as well as my physical self. That is a good thing; I just hope I can make it.

Life is hell. Life is not hell. Life is beautiful and I thank God for its beauty everyday. This is so drastic, I think I'm manic. My thoughts and feelings change from one second to the next. I'm losing my mind most days.

God, this disease does far worse things to your mind than it could ever do to your body. But, hopefully I will come out of it far more enlightened and in touch with my body and soul so as to live out the rest of my life truly healthy.

August 10, 1998

What did we come to learn?
What did we come to do?

Namaste – a soul to soul moment – translated it means: "The divinity in me beholds the divinity in thee." (It is a greeting to travelers passing each other in the Himalayas)

August 12, 1998

I barely slept all last night. I think I am stressed about the tests and scan tomorrow. I am also not feeling well. My stomach is extremely bloated.

One day at a time – one day at a time. Why do we have to look ahead? I must master meditation so as to master living in the moment and for the moment. Stop worrying – no longer allowed. It serves absolutely no purpose. Worrying is as useless as jealousy!!

Negative energy – where is all this negativity coming from? It is useless and serves no purpose in my life. I wish my emotional side could be as logical as my intellectual side!

Good luck to me tomorrow!!!!

August 16, 1998

I had the test about the status of the tumour done today and now can only wait. The whole weekend has been kind of testy. I'm walking on a tightrope. On one side there is life and some degree of happiness and on the other side is the underworld and all it brings with it.

I must get into a new headspace starting tomorrow to finish the last four weeks of this nutritional program. I've been cheating a lot. That must end. I feel like I'm in really big trouble here and I don't know how to get back on track.

August 19, 1998

I'm in shock. My scan showed that the tumour is BIGGER. After all that hard work it hasn't shrunk. The nutritionist can't believe it. I can't believe it. I'm running out of steam. I feel like I need to go away and eat and drink and contemplate life.

I can't write – here right now. I'm so tired.

August 24, 1998

I must come to terms with and accept that life, as I knew it, is over at least for awhile. My focus word is: Healing

I will talk to my Inner Child – ask what she needs to get well. I want to be my Inner Child's hero.

August 25, 1998

I'm sitting here waiting for the seaplane to go to my favorite place on Pender Island. I need to get away. I've been pretty fucked up since the results last week. I had a fantastic weekend off the metabolic program. I had such a great time feeling normal again. I can't help but wonder if that great time for my soul didn't do me as much good as the program. I will never regret doing it. I'm still having a very hard time following the program.

I think I'm still shocked at how this tumour is growing and God knows what else, even with everything I've been doing, physically and spiritually. I will have to go through another surgery to deal with the tumour and am determined to stay very strong for it. That's the weird thing – I feel so strong. I have started walking with positive reinforcements as I go. I am also doing sit ups every day to try and strengthen my stomach muscles for my surgery in three weeks.

> *My husband, Mack, and I have a cottage on Pender Island, in the Gulf Islands of British Columbia. It is a perfect place for a quiet getaway. Erin sometimes came to the cottage with me and other times visited on her own. She fell in love with the natural setting and it was a sanctuary for both of us. Together we practiced QiGong with the rising sun, energy treatments on the outside deck, and in the evenings, sat out with a beautiful palette of stars. Erin found she experienced a greater clarity about what was happening to and around her and learned how to just BE with herself and nature.*

August 27, 1998

I'm at the cottage on Pender Island feeling very relaxed and at peace. Healing work here is much different than healing work in the city. Alma is with me and we had our session out on the deck this morning. My sensations are very clear and my mind seems less cluttered here. It is easier to focus on what I want to accomplish.

I did good work today. I felt that for the last few days my bladder and cervix were very tight like a big knot, so we worked on releasing that. I felt that my bladder and cervix were frantic – looking for the parts of me that are no longer there.

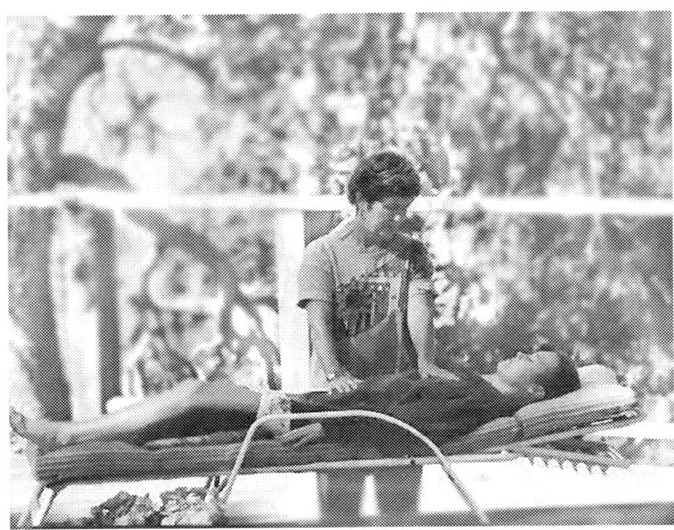

I feel that all of my abdominal organs are friends and when my uterus and ovaries were removed the other organs had to grieve the loss of their friends. I think my bladder and cervix were also afraid that they might be taken away in the next surgery, that's why they felt nervous. I tried to calm and re-assure them. I think it worked.

Also, there was some sadness in my heart that I wanted to hold onto. I felt my Inner Child/abdomen sad today but I allowed the feeling, gave it a hug and assured it that everything would be okay and like a child held in his mother's arms, the sadness lessened.

I visualized the tumour as a big knot of emotions that should have been released over the years but because I was so shut down, they just gathered in a knot.

Today I worked on unraveling that tumour and draining it out of my body to the point where I no longer saw a mass of any kind. My bladder relaxed and I tried to massage it into a larger capacity. I think it worked. I also filled my uterus and ovary area full of white light, in their shape, to maintain the internal energetic feeling for my other organs. I do feel whole. I am healthy.

I have been putting some thought towards slowing down on the program for now to build some strength for the surgery and it would be good for my mind. I'm also concerned about my low blood pressure. I can do little workouts and feel healthier.

September 7, 1998

Well, I'm embarrassed about how long it's been since I've written in this journal. I have been going a little crazy and enjoying life so much these last two weeks. I am still eating properly and taking some of the pills every day. I was extremely social last week and this week also. I feel rock solid strong. I am working out every morning and feeling really good for it. Everyone says I look really good. I do feel like I look great! I really like my short hair and am actually starting to feel like myself, my real self.

I know I have worked hard up to now, physically and spiritually and I believe God will smile on me.

Although I am scared shitless for surgery – not the operation itself, I think I am stronger and healthier than before the last surgery. There is no reason to think and expect that this won't be better, quicker to recover. But I am nervous to hear of what they will find. It's a fine line when faced with a situation like this to be optimistic yet realistic.

I am young and I am strong but I believe that part of beating this is also in a way spiritual destiny and a little luck. I know I have worked hard up to now, physically and spiritually and I believe God will smile on me. I have to be up and at the hospital early for pre-op stuff. I haven't been sleeping at all well and I'd like to try again tonight for me.

I'll be back soon.

September 11, 1998

THE HEALING HOUSE

I hardly know how to describe this. I am sitting in a piece of heaven. Tranquility, peace, joy, fulfillment and health are all around me here. I've come to the cottage on Pender Island for the weekend to get away by myself for a few days before surgery. There could not be a more healing place for me on this earth. I've felt it here from the first time I visited. My soul is at peace here, completely fulfilled. I see myself doing a lot of mental and physical healing here. I believe that the outdoors close to nature is where the most substantial healing can occur. Everything is so honest here, to the core.

Some things in our lives will happen to us because that is what is supposed to happen. The point is not what happens to us but how we handle it. And how we handle it is what determines what path we will ultimately go down.

I read my I Ching (a book of ancient Chinese wisdom – a system of changes) this afternoon. My question was: "What is it that will result from this period of deepening self awareness and deeper knowledge of self?"

Answers:

1. It is too soon to answer the 'results' question and it said to set limitations on my life in regards to finance and relationships. It said not to expend energy on others through this difficult time.
2. It reinforced the need for balance. I must not think about work or anything besides restoring healthy boundaries in my own person. It also said to watch excesses. Do not follow one path exclusively and to excess. Keep an open mind to various healing paths, incorporating them all in my life.

It was great to get this reading because it makes me feel that my gut instinct, the Universe, and all my psyches and powers are in sync. I am on the best track for my highest good.

Yes, situations can be ultimately very scary and negative but what are you going to do about it? Own your life and everything that comes with it – don't let a situation own you.

The basis for the I Ching is that we are all a part of the flow of this Universe and as such, we must flow, like water, with the Universal tide. Some things in our lives will happen to us because that is what is supposed to happen. The point is not what happens to us but how we handle it. And how we handle it is what determines what path we will ultimately go down.

I think that taking control of our situations gives us the upper hand in determining or deciding our fate or destiny. It is those that just let everything happen to them without exercising our God-given ability to think and feel and perceive, are the people that will die very badly. Bad things do not happen to good people (as the saying goes). I think negative things can happen to us in our lives but we choose what to do with them and what to learn from them. That is within our power as human beings.

Yes, situations can be ultimately very scary and negative but what are you going to do about it? Own your life and everything that comes with it – don't let a situation own you.

I believe, deep down, that I will be okay but from now on, as long or as short as it may be, this has been and is, the most incredible journey I have or will ever experience.

The mere action of owning the situation, as bad as it is, maybe just taking control of your own healing, your body's innate healing, understanding and abilities, can change an intolerable situation into one of fantastic enlightenment and learning. I have chosen that path for my journey. I believe, deep down, that I will be okay but from now on, as long or as short as it may be, this has been and is, the most incredible journey I have or will ever experience.

A more perfect night there couldn't be, sitting out on the deck. It started with a few stars in the sky. I thought to myself how beautiful the night is and then, as a thrill, a shooting star appeared in the sky. I made my wish. I felt like God had sent me the shooting star. Then the wind picked up a little, the clouds blew away and all the stars began to appear. The sky is now clear, full of stars and the Milky Way is apparent. I am so thankful to be able to experience this wonder, God's wondrous universe. We are here to appreciate it and be thankful for it. And I am.

I began to notice a new level of spirituality emerging in Erin. For the past nine months she explored Journal Writing, Healing Touch and Diet Detoxification, as purging tools to help her reveal her inner self – a buried treasure coming to light.

This new level of awakening was now more present in her journal writing as she talked about difficult experiences and profound insights relating to her new-found connection with her soul. Being so close to her, the associated growing pains were a mixed message for me because I was her therapist, and now a good friend. I felt joy for her new-found enlightenment but pain as I witnessed the cathartic process she endured in this journey.

"No one ascends from the underworld unmarked"

~ "Close to the Bone" by Jean Shinoda

CHAPTER 4

The Letter

"When I ask you to respect my needs – please do so."

~ Erin Higgins

October 2, 1998

This is a lonely battle once again. I know I haven't written in here for a long time since just before the surgery. That was such a wonderful weekend full of hope and anticipation for the results! "Difficult beginning" is what the I Ching called it. It could not be much harder than this. The results were odd.

Surgery was a breeze as far as major surgeries go. I will never forget waking up September 14th and SMILING! I had no pain like the first time and remember laughing to myself in recovery. I came out of the anesthetic very quickly. I remember reaching down to my left side and feeling the colostomy. My first thought was that they had been able to remove the tumour – that was the stipulation of the colostomy – it was only to be done if it meant removing the tumour. But was I wrong! I have a colostomy because my bowel was eventually going to cause obstruction. The tumour was virtually inoperable – to remove it, they would have to make a hole in my bladder, which they did not want to do.

The cancer itself, Dr. B. said, was nasty looking and aggressive. They actually believe that because it is a more aggressive type that the chemo will have a better chance at killing it. I imagine it like many Pac Man's in my stomach chomping it out!

That afternoon, after Dr. B. had told me the results and left, I proceeded to go into complete shock for at least one hour. Mom, Sylvia and Alma stayed with me to try and calm me down. It was a very weird and scary process. My arms and legs went completely numb to the point where my arms curled up onto my chest. Then, I had tightness in my chest; it felt like someone was standing right on me! I cried and cried and cried. I was in complete and utter shock. Hyperventilation – it was awful. It finally subsided and sleep came.

Then something happened. Call it SURVIVAL INSTINCT, but I just took a deep breath and said to myself "Okay what's the next step?" I can't do anything about the way it is now but I can't just let it happen! So you move on! Dad says I have this great ability to take my situation, whatever it may be and run with it. I don't know any other way to do it because anything else would just be giving up! And I can't in good conscience, allow that at this point. Maybe one day but not yet.

Then something happened. Call it survival instinct, but I just took a deep breath and said to myself "Okay what's the next step?" I can't do anything about the way it is now but I can't just let it happen! So you move on!

October 4, 1998

I met with the nutritionist today. I am going to continue on a program with him – a medium one, with no detox involved. I still believe in my heart and soul that the best thing I can do is a combination of chemo, metabolic therapy and energy healing.

October 5, 1998

My first time back at chemo was September 28th and right on schedule, my hair started to fall out. I don't know why it is bothering me so much. I've been through it before and you'd think after all the spiritual work I've been doing, it wouldn't bother me so much. I love myself and my friends and family love me, so why do I care if I have hair or not. I know that this is my spiritual journey and my appearance has nothing to do with it – it's all about what's inside. It's not about getting a date or primping my hair to go out. I know all that so why does it bother me so much?

I'm bald again! I had hoped to make it to Lara's wedding with hair but I already had bald patches so made an executive decision to shave it all off. So here I am looking like the cancer poster child once again.

I can't believe what a virtual non-issue the colostomy is. It is very easy to care for, all my supplies are paid for and it's really nice not to have to worry about constipation.

October 18, 1998

I had a cry on the way home from dinner at Mom's. I know I have gained incredible knowledge and spirituality and have really gotten to know myself but none of that can hold me at night. None of that can look into my eyes on my worst days and tell me I'm beautiful. Who the hell is going to want a bald, eyebrowless, eyelashless woman with a colostomy and foot long scar on her belly who can't have kids and is, chances are, if she's lucky, only going to live another three to five years? Sound like a good package to you? I think not.

October 31, 1998

Sometimes I just sit here and can't believe that the surgery was not more successful. I wonder how long it will be before I have problems physically due to the tumour. So far it's just the precautionary colostomy. That is a defeatist attitude I prefer not to allow into my thinking but I do acknowledge the thoughts are there! I have to.

I feel very unfocused. I felt so driven, focused and determined before surgery. I am still working to get that back – ever since I found out that the metabolic program didn't make the cancer better. I am still shocked about that. Now, I have just finished my second round of chemotherapy. I really did not think I would go back to chemo and I have had to mentally get myself back into it after having talked my way out of it. I hope and pray with everything in me that this works.

Another stressful issue is that Dr. P. has suggested not doing any supplements for three days around my chemo treatment. She says that heavy supplements tend to protect cells – bad ones included! As if I need this right now. So I don't know what to do! Who to listen to? I feel like I'm back to last March when I didn't know who to listen to or who to trust. Sometimes I really don't know if I'm equipped for this fight! I'm really tired of the course my life is on right now!

I'm bald again! I had hoped to make it to Lara's wedding with hair but I already had bald patches so made an executive decision to shave it all off. So here I am looking like the cancer poster child once again.

I'm going to Pender Island on Monday for a few days. I hope to return with some clarity, focus and renewed determination. I have a few questions for I Ching. God be with me – PLEASE!

November 2, 1998

I think about dying a lot, about my funeral, about writing out my last wishes for Lara to have. I feel very comfortable about the afterlife. I believe my soul will live on. It will go on to the next life it chooses. I just hope I learn all that I am supposed to in this life to make all of this worthwhile.

I write whatever comes to mind and that always seems to be current events. I know I should be writing about past events that I have 'issues' with but I feel like life now is too short to dwell on those. I have made peace with my past – so be it. I believe I have more stress now dealing with the financial worries and treatment strategies than any buried stress. I know I have days when I'm still pissed off at my ex and my lover and my stupidity but I think I always will. I have accepted the fact that my affair was the most passionate and exciting time of my life. I am deeply sorry for the hurt it caused but I don't regret a single moment of it. I was very in love. That is the truth – so be it.

I feel very comfortable about the afterlife. I believe my soul will live on. It will go on to the next life it chooses. I just hope I learn all that I am supposed to in this life to make all of this worthwhile.

When I'm here at Pender and I sit down and write and think about the adventures that could lie before me and I get excited. I feel the future is promising. I know I have a problem that, right now, makes me feel closed in and suffocated. It's not good and has to change. That's why I have escaped to here. I am craving direction, focus and a plan! I will have those when I leave here this time.

November 3, 1998

I'm too serious – too much pressure I put on myself. I worry about meditating enough, eating the right stuff, sleeping enough, exercising just right, appreciating nature enough etcetera, etcetera. It's way too much pressure. I have to learn to relax and just live: live well, live happy, listen to my body and my soul and do what they say.

I am learning so much through this journey and I am changing all the time. But with a large circle of awareness comes what feels like more pressure to incorporate all that I learn into my daily life. Not only because I am learning the importance of it, but there is the added pressure of feeling and thinking that it will help me conquer this disease. Knowledge and the accumulation of knowledge is wonderful but must be tempered with the understanding that you can't and don't necessarily have to, put it into practice all at once. Take one step at a time – one day at a time. Do not let the pressures mount.

I have to learn to relax and just live: live well, live happy, listen to my body and my soul and do what they say.

Do I journal enough, do I forgive enough, have I spent enough time closing relationship circles of the past? Is closing a circle necessarily finishing the issue? No, you have to acknowledge and resolve the feelings that go along with that circle. Release, Realign and Refocus – all for my highest good.

November 4, 1998

My primary responsibility is to myself and I am doing all I can do to heal my body of this disease. My secondary responsibility is to be one with the Universe that created my Forever Soul, and to use the knowledge I have acquired in this fight to help others in my situation.

I've renewed my focus to support my goals I had before surgery: to get back on the metabolic program, to exercise, to do my best with Alma, to do my best with chemo, to meditate even if only for five minutes, and to volunteer in the community. I feel good, deep inside, about these goals. I believe that it is my responsibility as a member of my community of family and friends to follow these goals. I also believe that it is my responsibility, as a soul that chose this life to be born into, is to try and learn as much as I can about this challenge and to share as much as I can about what I am learning. It is my responsibility to the Universe to do this before my soul moves on to its next chosen life.

My primary responsibility is to myself and I am doing all I can do to heal my body of this disease. My secondary responsibility is to be one with the Universe that created my Forever Soul, and to use the knowledge I have acquired in this fight to help others in my situation.

For the first time in weeks I feel like I know my purpose and focus. That is what I came to Pender to find and wouldn't you know after three days of thinking on it, asking I Ching about it and calling my Guides and Angels to help me with it, I think I figured it out! I promise to abandon my financial worries and questions of whether or not to move to a new apartment.

I will trust that the situations will present themselves to me, should the time come, when I must make changes.

For now I trust that the above commitment is for my highest good and all else in my life is progressing as it should, as it is meant to. From some of my reading these words have stayed with me:

"The Universe will never push you beyond that which you are ready for",
and
"Where you are is exactly where you need to be"

November 14, 1998

The Wedding

Lara and Steve's wedding created a beehive of activity and Erin was a major part of it. Her marketing contacts and experience were key factors in planning the whole event. She was front-and-centre all night and looked stunning in a low cut, indigo velvet gown with matching hat.

Mack and I, along with friends and relatives from across Canada shared the excitement that flowed throughout the evening. Lara said some people called it "Erin's Wedding" and Lara was pleased with that perception.

Erin shared love and humor in her toast to the Bride and Groom.

"I remember Lara and Steve's first date. I was at a local restaurant with a few friends and Lara dropped by and introduced her very shy, rosy-cheeked date named Steve. He barely said two words and I could tell he was quite intimidated by five loud, fairly rambunctious women inquiring about his background.

He seemed so quiet and shy I thought to myself "Oh God, someone that shy will never make it in this family!" But, as time went on I realized that that shyness transformed itself into a funny, warm, loving and caring person that I have come to love and value in my life very much.

If there is one thing that I think embodies their relationship it's that Steve and Lara are so in love – all the time. Their relationship has always seemed so special to me and I've had the opportunity to spend a lot of time with them, especially this last year. They have always been there for me and I have spent many, many nights in their spare bedroom. I find myself, especially these last few months, drawn to their house. I know when I'm there I am surrounded by love, understanding and so much laughter! That is one of the best things about these two – they are so funny together.

I know that I have been blessed with angels that have been sent to me in this life to help me through my challenges and Steve and Lara are definitely among them.

More seriously, they have been there for me at the drop of a hat, a moment's notice they climb into their car at 11 o'clock at night and drive 45 minutes to my house when I don't want to be alone, just to give me a hug.

I know that I have been blessed with angels that have been sent to me in this life to help me through my challenges and Steve and Lara are definitely among them."

November 25, 1998

I went to see Alma tonight with a liver and spleen that felt five times their original size. Everything from my rib cage down felt distended, sore with sharp pains.

When Alma began working on me she felt it right away. She worked away from my body and couldn't get past my fifth energy level. Every move she made with her hands caused serious discomfort and pains in my liver and spleen. We worked on clearing a lot of anger. Anger I felt towards men, family and friends. I worked on releasing, releasing, releasing and to my continued amazement it did get better. Since Lara's wedding I have been on automatic pilot and I think, no, I know, I have a lot of post-event stress and nerves. I partied late, repeating old behaviour patterns. Just writing about it makes my stomach turn. Situations and arguments with men in my life made me realize I was reverting back to my old ways and I paid for it.

I do not always speak my truth and it's gotten me into trouble. I/we all must speak our truth – always. One day at a time.

I CANNOT let that happen. It is such a long learning process. I am amazed that my physical pain was due to emotional baggage that I refused to let go of AGAIN. My one-day-at-a-time focus must return. I have to work on it harder. I have to work on me harder. I do not always speak my truth and it's gotten me into trouble. I/WE ALL MUST SPEAK OUR TRUTH – always. One day at a time.

November 27, 1998

My last entry in this journal is so appropriate for today! I wrote a letter to my family explaining to them how I feel. Dad is insisting on going to chemo with me on Monday even though I specifically asked him not to. I actually said to him "I don't want you to come." He replied that he was coming because he wants to stay "plugged in" to this whole thing. Also, he is insisting on giving me $1000 per month! I again told him that I do not want his money – that is why I am going back to work because I don't want any more money from him and Mom. Again, he does it anyway. I GIVE UP!

My stomach feels distended, swollen, tight, nervous, and anxious. I really feel like I'm a mess and just long to feel healthy again.

I'm very tired tonight. I'm going to go and meditate now.

The Letter

Dear Family,

I am writing this letter to try and explain to you how I am feeling, physically and mentally in the hopes that it will help you to understand why I ask for the things I do and why I make the choices that I make everyday. Anything I say in the next few pages is most definitely not meant to hurt, disappoint or push away any of you. I love you very much for your support and unconditional love and I think that this will only help you to know how to best help me.

When this whole battle first began the sense of loss was almost unbearable. I cried for the babies I would never have and actually felt like I missed them, even though I didn't know them. I cursed God for 'doing' this to me and honestly felt that it was some kind of payback for the affair I had when I was married. For me to sit and think about the incredible magnitude of all that I have lost is overwhelming, even to this day. I work very hard at coming to terms with all that I may never be able to do – either because of physical limitations or a possibility of running out of time. I think that is why I live as large and as hard as I do now. I can't afford not to.

After my first surgery, I pretty much blocked out all that was happening to me. I worked hard through my chemo to try and keep my life as intact as I could, all the while watching my hair fall out strand by beautiful strand. I still miss my long blond waves every day.

It has taken me until now to feel complete and to appreciate the wonderful me inside which is reflected outside.

This experience has made me realize how I have always been defined by my looks and physical appearance. I look at myself now – bald, colostomy and a scar dividing me in half and the person that I was is no more.

I feel, for lack of a better word, damaged. It has taken me until now to feel complete and to appreciate the wonderful me inside which is reflected outside. You have all helped me to do this, as have my friends and the very special men in my life. I do have my days when I ask myself if I am ever to be in love again – who could possibly want me? Not able to have kids – so scarred – yet these thoughts are few and far between. Rest assured that on the majority of days I feel excellent about myself.

I ground myself and fight from where I am, not wonder where I could or would be if …

Things came crashing down and reality set in when, last May, Dr. H. came into the chemo room and told me that it wasn't working. I was on the floor for a week. I couldn't wrap my mind around work anymore so I decided to leave it behind and focus on me.

Not a very difficult decision at the time although I would miss it a lot.

The metabolic/nutritional program was brutal and all consuming. I was convinced beyond a shadow of a doubt that I was getting better. When the scan in August revealed the opposite, my world came crashing down again. How much could one person take without going over the deep end? I absolutely don't regret doing those three months of that therapy but I would be lying if I said I didn't think about what would have been if ... but no time for that. I ground myself and fight from where I am, not wonder where I could or would be if ...

My fourth big crash was post–op September 14th. Could it have been any worse? I will never forget waking up from surgery that day and laughing to myself. I felt the colostomy and figured they had removed the tumour because those were my conditions of accepting a colostomy – only if it was to remove the tumour. I felt like someone was standing above me saying "Here, Erin, I'm going to kick you again and see if you can get up this time!" I ground myself once again, take stock of where I am and begin a new fight, from a new place, with new challenges.

I am so thankful for the body I have and amazed at how strong it remains in the face of so much dis-ease. I also strongly believe that our souls come back many times and each time we choose the body we will be born into in order for our souls to grow from the challenges that will be presented. I accept my challenges with zest. Although this experience is extremely interesting and exhausting, it is the life that I have and I refuse to waste it feeling sorry for myself. The sun still rises everyday and the world gets on to a new day of life, as do I, even though sometimes I wish it would just stop for awhile.

I have done a tremendous amount of 'soul' work since this began and I have come to know myself very well. I know what I need and what I don't need. I know what makes me truly happy and what gives me tremendous stress. I appreciate every second, whether I am laughing or crying. Most importantly, I have learned to speak my truth and that is why I am writing you this letter. You see, I have to speak my truth, all the time because if I don't it all gets stuck in my gut and helps the disease to grow.

I have done a tremendous amount of 'soul' work since this began and I have come to know myself very well. I know what I need and what I don't need.

That, I believe, is how it got there in the first place – years of lying to myself and to others about how I really feel and what I really need.

When I went to Pender Island last month, I felt very confused about how to handle my life. When I came back I was sure I had figured it out. My #1 priority should be to teach others what I have learned. So here I was with my priorities. I soon learned that what I needed to do to heal myself was not as time consuming as when I was on the nutritional program. I realized that what I need to do is be as genuinely happy as possible under the circumstances.

I realized that what I need to do is be as genuinely happy as possible under the circumstances.

I also realized that I could not go on any longer being financially supported by my parents. That in itself causes me more stress than going back to work would. I have to be able to go away, buy clothes, and go out without feeling a need to justify it to my parents. So after much soul searching and consideration, I went back to work. This decision was very difficult for me because I did not want to commit to Monks if I wouldn't be able to pull it off, but I decided that I could and would do whatever is necessary to make it work. The agreement I have with them is that three to four days a month, after chemo, I will not be there. There are no guarantees that I will be there in three months, or six months or six years but they are okay with that. I will do my best for as long as I can.

I will tell you now that I am working full time, that is the agreement. I have an assistant to work the two days per week that I will be out of the office doing outside sales. The month of December is extremely busy. I will be working six days a week, more if necessary.

I am telling you this now so that you are not surprised or upset or worried by my work habits. This is the way it is going to be and the way I want it to be so please do not tell me not to work too hard or to slow down because it is not going to happen. You must understand that although it is a stressful job it is good stress.

I worked my first function, since I came back, this weekend and it was exhilarating. I can't explain the immense satisfaction I get from the job. Not to mention how wonderful it feels to have the staff that I know tell me how great it is to have me back and the staff that I had not yet met tell me how great it is to work with me because they had heard great things about me.

Since the 'Wonderful Nightmare' (as I like to call it) began, I learned to work on my inner health and spirituality by doing a lot of visualization, meditation, and journal writing. I find these to be extremely powerful in their ability to make me feel strong and healthy. Because my days are very busy, I really enjoy using my chemotherapy time to meditate and write. This is also very important in the 'mental game' of helping the chemo to work. This is the reason that I prefer to go to chemo on my own. I really don't want anyone else there with me. I don't mean to shut any of you out or push you away but I ask you to please respect my wishes on this point. I feel very stressed with the doctor or in chemo if any of you are there. If you need to be there for your own reasons you will have to find a way to deal with that. With all due respect that is not my problem. I can only handle what is on my plate. I'm sorry that I can't help you deal with your issues too but I just can't. You have each other; use each other.

I really don't like it when you make a big deal out of the chemo day. It's just a visit with the doctor; there is never anything new and a few hours of intravenous. Please don't circle the days on your calendar. I don't, so why would you?

I have arranged with the agency that I will receive all my blood test results so if there is ever anything out of the ordinary I will tell you. Otherwise, everything is normal, or as to be expected. Chemo is going to be in my life for a long time so let's just incorporate it in. I am tired for four to five days after each treatment and I have traveling pains in my abdomen during that time. I'm also pretty cranky and not very talkative in that following week. I am telling you this so that you know how I feel. It doesn't change; it's the same each time. This is all just a normal part of my life now, very cyclic, very consistent. I don't want to make a special occasion every month warranting multiple phone calls per day and undue concern. It really drives me crazy. Just know that I am fine. It sucks but it's all very manageable.

This is my body, my health and my experience and you have to trust that I am doing my absolute best to be well.

I guess what I want you all to remember is that I'm a 32-year-old grown woman. I am strong, fiercely independent and extremely active. Please don't call me and ask what I'm having for dinner to check up on me. It's condescending and hurtful. It means to me that you don't trust me. This is my body, my health and my experience and you have to trust that I am doing my absolute best to be well. Yes, I know what it means to have fries instead of salad but I'm still going to choose the fries every now and then. And you must also understand that my conscience is clear about that choice.

Whether I die next month, next year, in ten years or when I'm eighty I will do it my way and it will be kicking and screaming.

Just so you know, I do take my vitamins, I eat well (not fanatically, but well), I have started working out again, I pray, I meditate, I see Alma, I work very hard and I socialize very hard and I thank God for each of you every day. That is my life. That is how I want it and that is how it will be. So please, when I ask you to respect my needs in this, please do. When you are doing something for me stop and really ask yourself if it is truly for me or is it to help yourself feel better. If the answer is that it is for you and it is at the expense of causing me stress, please don't do it. You have to remember that is my journey and as much as you want to be there for me or do it for me, you can't. I don't envy your position as family members at all; I think I would go crazy if it was one of you.

Please know that spiritually, emotionally and psychologically, I am healthier than I have ever been in my life.

Please know that spiritually, emotionally and psychologically, I am healthier than I have ever been in my life. I am very happy working hard and being very busy socially while still ensuring I spend quiet time for care of my soul. I have my bad, low days but that is par for the course. I deal with it as it comes up, with a lot of help from everyone around me.

I love you all very much and I hope this letter helps you to understand me better. Thanks for your support and patience.

Love,

Erin

XOXO

CHAPTER 5

I'm learning as fast as I can

"The Universe will never push you beyond what you are ready for"

December 23, 1998

This Christmas doesn't feel like Christmas. I have so much on my mind with being back to work and chemo and this dis-ease. I want to be healthy again. I want my hair back. I'm sick of this shit. Please, dear God, on this, your Son's birthday, rid me of this incredible burden – take away this pain. I pray for a spontaneous remission. Please, dear God, don't let this be my last Christmas.

December 26, 1998

I think about dying all the time. I think about living all the time. How completely fucked up all this is. Nothing makes sense anymore. Feelings come and go with every breath. Ideas, goals, wants, needs change with the wind and certainly with every new day. How does one maintain sanity in this perpetually confused and changing environment? I'm sure I don't know! The answer is there are no answers! We strive our whole lives to answer our perpetual, theological and philosophical questions only to find that in the end there are no answers! Only more questions. Why?

December 29, 1998

Today was a great day. My side (liver) is feeling better. I think it was mad at me because of the pace of work in December and too much partying! So I haven't been drinking at all, eating better and taking all my vitamins. I went for a run last night and felt very strong. It amazes me how I can have all these little aches and pains while sitting on the couch but when I go for a run, everything feels so clean and healthy. This week has been very relaxed at work, easy. I've been getting a lot of sleep. I love the quiet.

I have another scan tomorrow and I don't even care what it says anymore I just want it to be over so I don't have to think about it. I say I don't care because I believe it's all in how I feel – that's what counts. It's so hard to hear bad news. I always prepare myself to expect the worst so that if it's better news it's a bonus but if it's bad it's expected!

We strive our whole lives to answer our perpetual, theological and philosophical questions only to find that in the end there are no answers! Only more questions. Why?

I did a lot of releasing with Alma today. I'm having a real problem with certain people in my life that keep coming up whenever I work on releasing stress and negative issues – they are male issues. I realized that it is a control issue. I feel, in different situations, a power/control struggle with them and also a belittling issue when I feel that they are trying to control me. This is a battle also within me of my male versus female sides.

Today Alma asked me to go very deep and see what the root of this struggle was. I found that the source is not from this lifetime but from a past life. It was really cool to go there. I traveled (via my third eye) through a dark hole. She said to keep going to the other side and after awhile I came out into the light and saw a little girl working on a farm.

I saw a very dominant male figure, I think it was her father, doing nothing but being very stern and giving her orders. I saw no mother around. The feelings I had were that I was the little girl working on that farm in the late 1800s or early 1900s and I was tired and worked very hard. When Alma asked what my feelings were, the first thing that came up for me was that I felt unappreciated by this man. I went back to that place as me and hugged that little girl for a long time and told her I loved her and really appreciated all the work she did. I got the man (father?) to tell her she was doing a great job and that he was thankful she was there. I also told her that I would be here to hold her and love her whenever she needed me. This seemed to release a lot for me – even my left side felt better!

Regardless of the outcome, I'm having an incredible journey figuring it all out. I can't believe that people live their whole lives without ever experiencing any of this! It's really too bad and that is why I need to write a book.

I really feel like I experienced one of my past lives. I truly believe that much of our tension, fear and problems with issues in this life are caused by leftover unresolved issues from past lives. Slowly but surely I'm getting to my past lives in the hopes of getting rid of whatever is causing this dis-ease in my body.

Regardless of the outcome, I'm having an incredible journey figuring it all out. I can't believe that people live their whole lives without ever experiencing any of this! It's really too bad and that is why I need to write a book.

December 30, 1998

Pretty good visit at the agency today. Dr. H. says everything is relatively unchanged. I do need to move on to a different treatment though because I can become resistant. I will look at my options this weekend and sit with it for a while and see how I feel. I think I need another trip to Pender.

Wow, tomorrow is New Year's Eve! Part of me wants to wipe out 1998 and the other part is so in awe of all I have learned and the new people I now have in my life. I have learned so much that I am appreciative of. A part of me actually feels that I wouldn't change a thing for all I have learned. I don't think anyone could really understand that but I don't think anyone could possibly understand the depth of enlightenment and understanding I have reached so far this year

It frightens me to think of what lies ahead for me in 1999. I pray that it brings me health. I pray that someone somewhere in the world finds a cure for this but above all else I pray for happiness, fulfillment, and physical strength to live large. I have New Years resolutions and a niece/nephew to arrive in 1999. I can't wait! Please let me be here to do it all.

January 2, 1999

Pain is a physical manifestation of the growth of your soul!

The whole thing is actually my worst nightmare. I always remember saying that my worst fear is to have my body slowly die before my mind – to have your mind sharp as a tack and your body weakening around you. I can feel things changing. I have pain along my right ribs. I don't know what it is. I don't want to know what it is. I am fighting this with everything in me. I am running, working out, working, socializing, taking trips, basically not ever letting this illness be the reason that I don't do something that I want to do. I hate this. I really hate this. I would give anything not to have this dis-ease. I want to live so much. I just can't accept that I could die young. It's not an option. I won't allow it.

I'm working on being a lot more patient with Dad. I actually have arguments with him in my head that never happen with him. I love him so much. I know that I get uncomfortable around him because he makes me confront the cancer. Everyone else is pretty normal. But his hugs are intense! His looks are sad. He's all over me all the time with love and hugs and unfortunately, all this does is make me angry because it is a constant reminder of how much he is hurting. I just don't want to deal with it all the time. I know that I need another weekend away by myself.

Pain is a physical manifestation of the growth of your soul!

January 5, 1999

I'm afraid to start a new chemo program because I'm afraid it won't work, like the two previous ones, and then I'll have used up yet another in the very short list of treatments to help save my life. I don't look forward to anything too far down the road anymore. I am much more focused on the here and now. For instance, this weekend I'm looking forward to: phones off, in bed, eight movies, my journal, my books and lots of food. What an absolutely perfect weekend. I can't wait! I can't believe that this is now my idea of a perfect weekend! No socializing – just me. I've grown so much this year.

January 7, 1999

Alma worked miracles. I arrived at her place feeling very short tempered, impatient, and extremely bloated. I felt like I was retaining water or something. While Alma was doing an energetic scan she found things quite heavy. She did a lymphatic drain and

I could not believe how much better I felt. It was amazing and I have not returned to that state since. Awesome!! I'm so lucky to have her – she is absolutely amazing.

January 11, 1999

I went to see Alma today before going to work. What a great session. I have been having a fair amount of discomfort on my right side – liver up to my ribs. Today, instead of doing hands-on work directly on the liver, Alma did a reverse spiral meditation. The object of this is to open you up so that all the spirals at each chakra are open and spinning out, to gather Universal energy. We found my third chakra blocked, which is the one that feeds my liver and heart. We worked to unblock it by releasing fear (that is what came up for me). Fear of starting a new program. That was released after a bit of time – it was difficult to get rid of. After its release I felt like I had been peeled open lying on the table.

I felt that all my energy centres were very open to information from the Universe to help me make my treatment decisions. It was a very odd feeling. I actually felt like I was lying there on the table and I was naked inside, completely open, split down the middle and peeled back, accepting everything my Guides and Angels wanted me to have. After that was done Alma 'closed' all the chakras and put the spirals back to their normal state. My side felt better. I felt very light, no stress, very go-with-the-flow. All day I have felt very relaxed. My side continues to feel great, even when I breathe deeply.

> *I learned to allow extra time in my schedule for Erin's sessions. In my treatment room in Richmond, or on Pender Island, Erin could say anything and be anything without having to prove anything. It was a place, away from her daily life, that she had the freedom to explore newly discovered territory. I was a therapist, not family, and there was an implicit code of confidentiality that created sacred space for her.*

With each treatment the bond of trust between Erin and me grew stronger.

Erin was insatiable in her learning and she remembered all the details of each treatment – something I wasn't used to with others. This attention to detail was reinforced for me as I read how accurately she wrote about her experiences in her journals in order to share what she learned with others.

January 17, 1999

Round 4!

I get up, I walk, I fall down
I get up, I walk, I fall down
Meanwhile I keep dancing…

That is my motto through this whole experience until it's over, until I am well again. Life goes on. Life must go on as normally as possible in order for me to maintain some sanity.

I feel nervous, almost anxious. I'm nervous about starting new chemo. I feel like I'm up against a wall. I hate being told what to do – by anyone, even myself! I long to be free. This regime is a nightmare. But through it all, most of me loves my life! It's very full and fulfilling. I will carry this time with me always, even once I am well again. I will never forget how I feel, trials and tribulations, successes and challenges. It was the best of times; it was the worst of times…

I can't wait till summer – failure is not an option.

January 18, 1999

This dis-ease is everywhere – something is terribly wrong with our world, our environment. There are just too many people with cancer.

It's still so surreal to me sometimes. I feel it but I don't feel it. I know it but I don't know it. I definitely hurt more than ever before but I try to ignore it. I rest when I need to but otherwise I just refuse to give it power.

January 20, 1999

I just finished listening to two tapes by Caroline Myss called "Why People Don't Heal". It was extremely interesting and thought provoking. In a nutshell she believes that we leave pieces of our soul at different situations in our lives when we have felt hurt and betrayed. We have a tendency to hold on to old hurts and wounds, never letting them go. What we must do is call our spirit back from all those places, forgive the people we feel did us wrong, all the while realizing that we choose to be hurt by their actions. We could have taken on a different perspective and choose not to be hurt by them, and in the forgiveness, call our spirit back. In doing that with all these situations, we end up with our whole spirit back and can live in the present. We must live in the moment, today, not thinking about the past or the future and be soulful.

It's still so surreal to me sometimes. I feel it but I don't feel it. I know it but I don't know it. I definitely hurt more than ever before but I try to ignore it. I rest when I need to but otherwise I just refuse to give it power.

By living this way, we will not leave pieces of ourselves anywhere else and with a complete soul can command it to change our biology to reflect health. As Carolyn Myss says "To know your biology, look at your biography".

What a revelation!! How freeing that is! Life is a spiritual journey and it's not about 'who did what to whom' – it's about spiritual growth and the lessons we (the Universe) have chosen to teach our souls. We choose the lives we are born into so that our souls will continue to learn and grow. So we should not take personally the things that happen to us in this lifetime because it is all for the growth of our spirit. It has nothing to do with us. That is what Caroline Myss meant when she said that life would be just a joy to live if we didn't take it personally!! We must distance ourselves emotionally from situations and accept growth and MOVE ON. Everything's a lesson and if we learn it right the first time we will never have to repeat it, in this life or any other!

What a revelation!! How freeing that is! Life is a spiritual journey and it's not about 'who did what to whom' – it's about spiritual growth and the lessons we (the Universe) have chosen to teach our souls.

January 21, 1999

When I got to Alma's tonight I felt like I was in pieces – my head here, my foot over there, my liver over there – so she put me back together. Even though my energy was excellent, all chakras looking good, I was exhausted. TOO MUCH INFORMATION when trying to make my next decision.

We did some releasing at my second chakra and then worked on my head! I love it when she works on my neck and head, it's so relaxing! Anyway I just wanted to write about a cool visualization exercise we did. She held my feet and we ran different colours into me, one at a time, from my feet up to my head. It was to work on my intuitive female side. When she suggested green and I imagined the green energy running up my body, my first intuitive feelings were cool and relaxing. Then we did red, this brought up busy, powerful and aggressive sensations.

No matter what you look like physically, just look into your eyes and see your soul and recognize that although your physical body may be changing, the beautiful you still resides inside.

Basically, this exercise teaches me how to use my female intuitive side – the emotional, creative side – rather then my male or analytical side. So now, when I want to relax, I can visualize green liquid running in me and when I need to feel powerful, I can run red liquid up my body. Really cool!

Erin arrived today feeling scattered, drained and just plain out-of- sorts. We did some clearing and clean up work on these scattered areas then decided it was time to play and go to 'Spiritual Kindergarten'. This concept is meant to make things simple and playful as you work with energy. Using colours and sensations Erin learned to move energy through her body. She realized how easy it was to do it herself and how it gave her a new awareness and level of control.

January 23, 1999

I was just watching a TV show the other day that showed a live cancer support group meeting. It validated my reasons for not going to support groups. I listened while a bunch of women sat around talking about their struggles, of which I admit there are many in this journey. One woman stated that she was on chemo, had been for two years, and when she looked in the mirror she didn't see herself anymore because of the hair loss, no eyebrows, baldness etcetera.

Leave what is in the past in the past and grow today, as the person that you have become instead of carrying your wounds in your back pocket for life – pulling them out whenever you need an excuse for something in your behaviour or development.

I got angry as all the women nodded "yes" to these feelings. I thought to myself how sad it was that these women are just not learning one of the most important lessons to come out of battles like these – IT IS YOU!!

They were still defining themselves by physical appearance instead of their soul. No matter what you look like physically, just look into your eyes and see your soul and recognize that although your physical body may be changing, the beautiful you still resides inside. If one doesn't see that, then you are a lost soul on this journey where soul is so important. We live in a world that defines us by our physical appearance and when dealing with a dis-ease that can take away some or all of your favourite physical assets, a healthy strong soul is so important. This is why caring for your spiritual and emotional self is more important almost than your physical self because they are what will get you through the times when your physical self may be falling apart or slowly fighting for its life!

Support groups, I find, tend to focus on what cancer patients have lost instead of what can be gained on this most incredible journey! So many of groups like AA and drug rehabs teach the survivor to hold onto their wounds and use them as a crutch instead of teaching them how to heal their problems. Leave what is in the past in the past and grow today, as the person that you have become instead of carrying your wounds in your back pocket for life – pulling them out whenever you need an excuse for something in your behaviour or development. That is why people go to 12-step programs for life, never really putting the addiction behind them and moving on with life in the present!

February 1, 1999

Lara started spotting this weekend and found out today that there is no baby in her womb! My first thought was to curse the Universe or God or whoever. Can't we have one positive thing happen in the family? I had a lot of anger and frustration but then I thought that when it is meant to be it will be.

February 9, 1999

I couldn't let this day go by without writing about it. Happy Anniversary to me! I can't believe that it has been one year today since all of this nightmare/wondrous experience began. It is a little overwhelming. In many ways I am healthier today than I was a year ago and yet I still have so much disease in me! So how did I mark this day? I worked from 10:00am to 8:00pm, came home, had a long hot shower and climbed into bed and began planning. I want to start writing a book about what my life has become and I have the inspiration to do it! I feel like it's a big step but I'm feeling strong and plan on remaining that way.

I'm so active it's unreal and yet I still spend a lot of quality time by myself. I think I have found an excellent balance and wish for an opportunity to live out a long and prosperous life.

As Alma said today, I've grown twenty years in the last year. I am very in tune with my body, I try to be good to it and respect it. I guess I am hoping it will return the favour to me and heal itself. This battle has just begun.

February 13, 1999

I feel angry about support groups for some reason. A friend told me she went to one a few days ago and it was awful – full of whining and crying and the facilitators never cut in, they just let it go on and on! Don't they understand that all the whining is just perpetuating the disease? Why is it that these women think that by sitting with a bunch of people they don't even know, that the others could understand what they are going through? Everyone deals with this differently.

Everyone has their own soul, their own level of understanding and self confidence. For example, how can I understand what someone I don't even know is going through? I can empathize, I can sympathize, but I don't know – the same way that no one on this earth can possibly understand what I'm going through because no one out there is me!! To truly understand what I am going through you would have to be me.

Support groups give cancer more power than it deserves. By whining and complaining you are allowing the cancer to run your life. Don't let it. You run your life, not the cancer!

I think that you truly get the best support from your friends and family because they are the people who most closely know your soul, your strengths, and your weaknesses. You just have to keep trying to explain things to them until they get it! That is your support – that and your own work at being soulful, growing every day and working on getting the mind-spiritual-emotional-physical connection happening that will make you complete and healthy. That my friends, is true support!

Support groups give cancer more power than it deserves. By whining and complaining you are allowing the cancer to run your life. Don't let it. You run your life, not the cancer! Why would anyone want someone to really understand their cancer journey? That would mean that they were in the same situation as you and I wouldn't wish that on my worst enemy.

I look at my family and friends and think, thank God you can't understand! Because if you did you would be where I am and I would never want that.

Support groups should be filled with positive healing energy zipping around the room. Let's talk about the wonderful closeness you felt with your daughter the other day or the special talk that you shared with your parents or how this disease has brought you to a new level of consciousness and spirituality that you never thought possible! Or how beautiful and vibrant colours look now and how great food tastes or how fresh the air smells! That is the stuff that others can't imagine. That is also stuff that your friends and family can't relate to – why not talk about that?

Support groups should be filled with positive healing energy zipping around the room.

<u>February 15, 1999</u>

Oh Happy day!!! I went to see Dr. H. today and he says I am responding to the chemo.

My pain around my liver and ribs is gone and he believes that the pain was definitely cancer-related. I am responding very quickly and he had thought it would take two months before we saw any improvement. I am very cautiously optimistic.

Excerpts from, *Mutant Message Down Under* by Marlo Morgan:

> **"..........when a doctor tells a patient there is no cure, that really means, in the doctor's education and background there is no information available to use for a cure. It doesn't mean there is no cure. If any other person has ever overcome the same disorder, then the human body obviously has the capability to heal."**

"Healing has absolutely nothing to do with time. Both healing and disease take place in an instant." ....."The Real People Tribe believes that we are not random victims of ill health. That the physical body is the only means our higher level of eternal consciousness has to communicate with our personality consciousness. Slowing down the body allows one to really look around and analyze the important wounds we need to mend: wounded relationships, gaping holes in our belief system, walled up tumors of fear, corroding faith in our Creator, hardened emotions of unforgiveness, etc."

I truly believe in what is written above. More than just believing it, I feel it deep in my gut. The more emotional garbage, Alma and I unfold, the better I feel – kudos to me!!

February 28, 1999

What is it that makes me (us) so insatiable in life? It's never enough! I always want more; need more to feel alive and fulfilled. It's not really 'the grass is always greener' syndrome because I don't look at other people and wish I had what they have (except for health!).

I have a great life – a great job, make good money, and am always going somewhere. I think I have the whole 'Carpe Diem' down pat but it's ultimately not enough. I need a new challenge. I'm not clear yet what it is I am here to do but I believe that cancer, as part of my journey, has put me on this road to find a way to help others.

March 6, 1999

I feel compelled to write about the last three days – the worst three days of my life! On Wednesday afternoon I left work early because of stomach pains and they got worse and worse as time went on. I ended up going to emergency where my two-day nightmare began.

I need a new challenge. I'm not clear yet what it is I am here to do but I believe that cancer, as part of my journey, has put me on this road to find a way to help others.

The x-rays showed a very large, distended stomach apparently a blockage or partial blockage in my intestine was to blame. The only thing to do was put an NG tube down my nose and into my stomach and pump out the contents.

The tube was undoubtedly the most imposing, uncomfortable thing I have ever experienced! The initial insertion through my nose was painful then the gagging began when the tube hit the throat area and I gagged all the way down to my stomach. Absolutely horrendous!

The rest of Wednesday night wasn't too bad. I had enough morphine and demerol to keep me out of it. Then my throat began to hurt and my sinuses were inflamed to the point my teeth were hurting! It was horrendous. I had to beg the doctor to take the tube out.

> *From the Emergency Ward, Erin's friends called and told me Erin wanted help with the pain. They asked if I would come. I was entertaining dinner guests and had drank a couple glasses of wine. I couldn't go to her and it tugged at my heart. That was when I realized how closely connected we had become and I knew her unknown journey was also mine.*

Mom and Alma were here on Friday and spent most of the afternoon holding cold compresses on my face to try and relieve the pain. By then I was drinking liquids and having no negative effects so the nurse took the tube out. As soon as it was out, relief set in. It was the most amazing feeling to have that thing out!

March 12, 1999

Writing is like exorcism I heard someone say in a movie. It can be. Sometimes I write because I hope the truth of my soul will come out, something subconscious will be exposed. Sometimes I write because I'm angry. Sometimes I write because I am lost. And sometimes I write because there is good news.

Sometimes I write because I hope the truth of my soul will come out, something subconscious will be exposed. Sometimes I write because I'm angry. Sometimes I write because I am lost. And sometimes I write because there is good news.

I am living and yet not. I am happy and yet not. I am fulfilled and yet not. I have direction and yet I do not. Life is getting complicated. All actions and feelings seem to have alternative subliminal meanings. Everything is suspect. I know I must change the path I'm on, I know that although I love my job it is not what I am to do in this lifetime. I must teach and influence those who need help in a more direct way.

I'm going to work everyday and loving most of it but not having energy left to do anything else. My purpose on this earth is bigger than that – I'm just not sure exactly what it is and how to find it. I pray that my Angels and Guides will help to show me the way. I am looking for signs of change: what to change, how to change, when to change. I feel it in my bones that I am not fulfilling my destiny and that is why I am always feeling stifled, frustrated and lost these past weeks.

I love everyone in my life but I feel I am growing past them. Maybe that is one reason that my inclination to do anything social is currently non-existent. I feel very cynical and sarcastic toward everyone right now – their simple uncomplicated lives with their little problems and little crises. They know nothing of crises.

When someone says "But my problem is nothing, I feel ridiculous even bringing it up to you" and I reply "No its okay, it's all relative to our own personal lives" – it's not okay. They are stupid little problems in relation to what could happen to you so buck up and deal with it! That's what I feel like saying but I don't because I remember when my problems used to be that small and petty. How I long for those days back!

So what is my road, my purpose in this life? It certainly isn't just to get cancer. I am on this road for a reason but I feel I've reached a fork in the road and don't know which way to turn. I either stay at a job I love and try to work in my writing and teaching or I leave work and travel and pursue writing a book and lecturing on 'the strength of the soul in the face of tragedy'.

March 14, 1999

Dissolving patterns dissolve disease, according to Louise Hay. She believes that healing cancer is like healing the mind – one must resolve old issues and clear blockages in order to dissolve the disease that has become the physical manifestation of these problems.

March 18, 1999

I feel like shit. My stomach problems have returned with a vengeance this week. Is this it? Is it downhill from here? I can't believe that it would be. I pray that it's not. My right side is starting to hurt again. My stomach hurts. My intestines hurt. My head hurts. I am miserable I can't get enough food in me to sustain energy. I don't understand why this is happening to me.

I look within, waiting for my body to speak to me and tell me what it needs. I actually do see the cancer getting smaller and going away. I feel like these problems are from scar tissue. I also feel that my intestines/bowels are tired and fed up with having to work so hard.

It is amazing to think of all the shit I have been through in my young life! From the time I was 20 things went from bad to worse to here – the ultimate hell.

March 20,1999

Caroline Myss says:

> "Divine justice and timing is perfect. We must understand this in order to live better and easier. Why am I dying? No earthly logic can explain this. Heaven does not live according to human justice. Our biography

> becomes our biology. We create our own reality therefore there can be no victims"

Buddha says:

> "There is nothing in the physical world that is stronger than you are, unless you give it the power."

March 21,1999

One of my friends, Karyn, is using me as a 'project' to create a video presentation for her journaling course. We began filming today. It took two hours of raw footage for a four minute presentation.

That gave me some time to really think about what it was I wanted to say and speak to. What was the 'truth' I wanted to pass on?

If any of you were part of such a project and had to focus on what you really believed in I think you would find it difficult. I know I did and I also know if I was part of the same project two years earlier my thoughts would have been totally different.

This data is taken from Erin's words on the raw footage of the video. For excerpts from the video, please see www.MyWonderfulNightmare.com

---

I have my own opinions about illness, specifically cancer but sometimes it's hard to define how things should be told. There are so many varying and outlying factors that are different for all of us.

The fact that I am now faced with a disease with life-changing consequences makes me look at everything differently. Most importantly, I now wake up each day and thank God for being here. I am learning to take one day at a time and enjoy each moment.

I believe it is important to our well being to learn to listen to our inner voice. That is one thing that is true and honest and something no one can take away from us.

We've never been taught to listen to our body and it's tragic. I somehow knew the results of my surgery before they told me. If I had been more in tune with my body I would have known earlier. I hadn't paid attention and didn't know how. If your body is telling you something is not right, ask for tests, look into it and don't be brushed off. Don't let doctors tell you nothing is wrong. Be aggressive with them – take control. When things bothered me three to four years ago it could have made a difference to my outcome if they had been dealt with then.

We've never been taught to listen to our body and it's tragic. I somehow knew the results of surgery before they told me. If I had been more in tune with my body I would have known earlier. I hadn't paid attention and didn't know how.

It's important to learn 'how' to listen to your body. The only way it has of talking to you is through sensations, pain and eventually disease. Listening to the body is basically using your intuition. It's something we all have but is a sense that is not honoured, valued and encouraged in our Western society. My heartfelt recommendation is to make a plan to develop that valuable tool.

My energy worker has told me, intuition is the 'first thought' that comes to you in response to an issue, that gut feeling. We usually try to think it over, rationalize it, judge it and by then most often we don't pay attention to it. So slow down and allow 'first thoughts and feelings' to have the value they deserve.

Another point I want to make is your right to get a second or third opinion if you don't believe you are being listened to. Sometimes a doctor may not pay attention to what you are 'really saying' and it's up to you to find one who will. We have the right to take control and make our own choices.

I knew it was important to become involved with every decision that affected my life. I had always been one to be in control but over the last several years I took a back seat to my husband and allowed him to control me. I knew I had to take that control back and I did. I learned from that and now refuse to be a victim without a fight.

My personal opinion is that it's paramount you understand that no one is going to cure you without your involvement. You need to do research, read and investigate yourself in order to understand what is best for you.

I hope to help others through this awareness of self-empowerment. I now have an opportunity to make a difference in my life as well as others if I use and share the tools I have been granted through my own experiences. In short – take control of The Beast – the illness and its related journey. It gives you power in your life when so much is being taken away from you.

In short – take control of The Beast – the illness and its related journey. It gives you power in your life when so much is being taken away from you.

I've been through two surgeries, three chemo treatments, three months of nutritional medicine, wear a colostomy bag and still follow my motto: I get up, I walk, I fall down and meanwhile I keep dancing. It seems beyond anyone else's comprehension to think my life goes on but it does. I still go to work because I love it and if it inspires me, then it is good for my immune system.

Last but not least, is the value of support and love from family and friends. These relationships have reached depths I never thought were possible for them or me in ways I couldn't have imagined. I also know I've enlightened them as well as myself through my journey.

Knowing what I know today, I don't think I would change a thing. This awesome experience of love and friendship has been an amazing, unexpected part of my journey. It actually has made it become 'My Wonderful Nightmare' – the perfect name for the book I plan to write.

Knowing what I know today, I don't think I would change a thing. This awesome experience of love and friendship has been an amazing, unexpected part of my journey. It actually has made it become 'My Wonderful Nightmare' – the perfect name for the book I plan to write.

May 12, 1999

I took a break and went away for awhile but traveling was hard on me. I am obsessed – obsessed with my stomach, obsessed with my anger, obsessed with feeling better, obsessed with every little ache and pain I feel. This can't be good. It is getting harder and harder for me to relax.

But there must be a way for me to live outside the hospital relatively pain free. I might try smoking pot for the pain to see if that helps.

I have such a hard time accepting pain management as opposed to actually solving the problem that's causing the pain. I have to accept that solving the problem may take a very long time and that pain management is necessary in the meantime. I want to do whatever I need to do to be pain free so that I can enjoy my days and do things instead of spending the day in bed in pain.

Okay! I just had a few tokes to see if pot would help my stomach. I did not enjoy the smoking – it made me cough and my chest burns! Lovely! Then I am stoned. My pain is still there. I just feel removed from it and it makes me eat and eat and I'm not sure this is helping the situation!

Okay! I just had a few tokes to see if pot would help my stomach. I did not enjoy the smoking – it made me cough and my chest burns! Lovely! Then I am stoned. My pain is still there. I just feel removed from it and it makes me eat and eat and I'm not sure this is helping the situation!

May 19, 1999

I've been thinking about dying a lot lately and whether it's my time or not. I'm not sure if I've made my mark in this world or still have yet to make it.

I'm not sure if we can even know if its our time until we are literally at death's door, minutes away and something kicks in to our subconscious and says either "Yes you can go now" or "No you can't" and the 'will to live' kicks in.

I have been told since this fight with cancer began that having a will to live is vitally important in my prognosis but of course I have a will to live! I am only thirty-two years old and have never had kids, look forward to grandkids, look forward to a healthy relationship, look forward to growing old with someone, would like to outlive my grandparents and parents, and I think that's only natural. Lara needs me in this pregnancy with a new baby and how could I not be here for her? Of course I have a will to live but is it helping me? I don't know.

We must never assume that the best place for a soul is among the living for that may not be. I believe it's up to the individual to decide and they should be supported in that wish.

Wait – I just got back from a walk and have to stretch – I'll be right back.

Okay, I'm back. I know I've been thinking about death and dying a lot lately because I feel like I've lost so much ground. I have lost about 20 pounds in two months and feel like a shadow of my former self. I'm tired all the time and I obviously have trouble eating. I have been in the hospital three times since February and it is not getting any easier to manage – only harder. The doctors say I need chemo again to stunt the growth of these new irritations on my small bowel that are preventing it from digesting food.

Unfortunately, I seem to have run the gamut of available chemos and none have worked for me. I am now into the study group of new treatments with no way of knowing whether they will work or whether I can get into one of the groups. For me, someone who believes in 'what will be, will be,' it is hard not to think that maybe the lack of success in treatments for me means that my time has come.

When I get tired and down I do think of the way my Nana went – peacefully, lots of morphine, sleeping at home. That is how I would want it to be. It's a type of suicide in a way, I guess, just choosing not to undergo any more treatments, doctors, and procedures. I find the option calming, actually.

Everyone has a different idea of what strength and life and soulfulness is. To some it is living life as fully as possible and to others it may be eternal peace and rest where the soul is free to do and be where it wants to be – healthy, strong and happy. We must never assume that the best place for a soul is among the living for that may not be. I believe it's up to the individual to decide and they should be supported in that wish. And to those who do not support the choice, I believe if they look hard enough in their own hearts and souls they will see that it is more for selfish reasons that they may want that person around, than for the dying friend they are losing.

May 28, 1999

Its 4:40 am and my mind is buzzing; sleep is lost. I have had relaxation tapes on for an hour but apparently sleep is not to be. I am tired but my mind races! I just found a new apartment and will be moving next week. I'm already stressed about having Dad here to help me – worried about what are you eating, when, why, are you okay, let me do this and that – but I know I am being ridiculous. It will be terrific to have his help. I wouldn't feel so stressed if it weren't for my own guilt about these things. I know I am eating whatever goes down and creates the least pain, whatever it is, chips, ice cream, anything that will give me some strength and pleasure.

My eyes are tired. They long for rest but my mind races on. Lists being made in my head of who I need to call to arrange the details of moving. It's the control side of me – I also honestly love doing it! It stresses me out but it's a positive high energy stress and doesn't feel negative, just tiring. But I do trust that my body and mind will sleep if they need to and it's not like I have to worry about work every day. I am my own project.

I'm leaving for Pender with Alma this morning for four days so I'll get plenty of therapy there! Well … I'm off to make lists in the absence of sleep!

> *We had a quiet weekend and worked mainly on relieving Erin's pain by pulling it from her body and replacing it with healing energy. The treatments took on a simpler approach. Deeper work of growth and enlightenment was no longer what she needed as it was too hard on her physically and so much of her soul work had been completed. Erin had a lot of other issues to think about now so we spent time in nature just talking, relaxing and simply 'being'.*
>
> *Erin didn't write in her journals about any further treatments but I did see her therapeutically in her home and in the hospital when possible, up to the last month of her life. Our work spanned two-and-a-half years; longer and more profound than I had ever experienced before and something I'll always carry in my heart.*

June 27, 1999

I remember when I was working full time, I would sometimes get so tired that I would 'see white' and 'feel white' – what is all that about? Absolute physical, mental and emotional exhaustion to the point of body shut down. It's like a cold 'sweet death' feeling.

June 28, 1999

I'm at the cancer agency for blood work, a doctor's appointment and a second round of chemo. I was just noticing how this disease targets everyone! A young Asian girl about 20 years old just came in. As I look around waiting room after waiting room in this building, I see how cancer crosses all income, generation, nationality, sex and any other line you could possibility imagine.

I haven't done much writing this last month. I haven't been able to. I have preferred to lose myself in trash novels so I can just stop thinking for awhile. Stomach problems have been off and on with two more hospital visits for the NG tube, a dose of steroids and a pain patch. So now I am playing with steroid dosages myself. Maintenance is the key. Eating is not bad. Good days and bad days. Up and down as always.

I'm so sick of waiting for doctors. I will never understand how, even if I am the doctors first patient in the morning, I can still be kept waiting. It's the fear and anxiety that makes this whole process so much more difficult.

TAKE CONTROL of your treatment, your situation, and your doctors. Ask questions, know how you feel and don't ignore those feelings. If something doesn't feel right, ask, cancel, or change your path. If you feel like you've been kept waiting long enough raise a fuss – NEVER STAY SILENT!

June 30, 1999

I started going to the Centre for Integrated Healing today. It's an alternative centre with multiple forms of therapy including 714x shots to boost the immune system, support groups and acupuncture. I just got back from my support group. I really enjoy the visualizations, art therapy and affirmation therapy.

I'm really tired today and yesterday, more mentally than physically. I am very lackadaisical, unmotivated, staring at daytime TV and frustrated by how stupid and unwatchable it is yet unable to motivate myself to do anything else. But there always seems to be something to do in maintenance of this disease.

Today and tomorrow is chemo and 714x shots and blood tests and stuff, stuff. I have officially, for right now, run out of patience with respect to needles, the cancer agency, bureaucracy, eating, medications and virtually everything that has to do with managing this disease.

I think about the women in my support group with Dr. G. and it just occurred to me that they all have children to take care of! Young ones! Their stresses are so much beyond mine. I just look after me. It is so wonderful that my friends and family have taken away all stresses in my life to leave me with just having to deal with my own situation but now I have nothing to distract me or anyone to need me.

Take control of your treatment, your situation, and your doctors. Ask questions, know how you feel and don't ignore those feelings. If something doesn't feel right, ask, cancel, or change your path. If you feel like you've been kept waiting long enough raise a fuss – never stay silent!

What a strange feeling it is turning out to be, to have no responsibilities beyond getting well. Not that that is not extremely high maintenance because it is, but it is just occurring to me that beyond me, there is no one relying on me for anything right now except love and friendship to my family and friends. WEIRD FEELING.

I feel inundated with this disease and maybe that is how it should be but I realize that virtually everything I do and think about everyday is me and I'm getting sick of it. I love what I am learning about me and soulfulness and mindfulness. The problem, however, is becoming that I don't read the books I want to because I'm sick of thinking about it. I don't do the cleansing that Alma and I talk about because I'm sick of it.

I write only in spurts now, waiting to begin putting a book together, but it's not starting because most of the time I'm sick of it! It is an odd paradox because although I am sick of it, I am enjoying this writing, as it happens. Maybe it's like working out – you never want to start but when it's over you're glad you did it … I think that's all for now, time to sleep.

P.S. No chemo side effects – Thank You!

CHAPTER 6

A Game with No Rules

"First God throws pebbles at you, then He throws a brick"

October 30, 1999

I haven't put pen to paper in months. I have not felt inclined to, nor inspired in any way. This last surgery almost 'killed me'. It was a big question for me and my family whether or not I should even have the surgery. I wasn't ready to throw in the towel. There was still some 'hope' within me and I believe we all need hope of some kind. Although all has worked out remarkably well, it has also taken from me things I am having a hard time getting back, such as spirit, PURPOSE, reason for being, etcetera.

I feel close to finding my purpose again. My niece/nephew-to-be is providing me with much incentive to begin new projects. I must begin my writing – short stories, chapters, letters to my niece/nephew, MY BOOK. Everyday I will commit one hour, at least, to writing. It may be one sentence or several pages but it must be something. This is my purpose. This is my new job! I must give back to this wonderful life and world. I

This is my purpose. This is my new job! I must give back to this wonderful life and world. I want to give back. And I am in desperate need of purpose right now in my life.

want to give back. And I am in desperate need of purpose right now in my life.

I spend my days fairly secluded in front of the TV looking forward to my next shot of the pain medication that I have become addicted to. I have told everyone about this addiction but no one seems to think much of it, or care, so I won't either. I know it's not right but I suppose if this is the worst thing I have right now it really doesn't matter.

The rain has arrived and with it, rebirth. The rain, the new baby, regrowth, all of this must bring with it hope for newness, new PURPOSE. I do believe that it is, to write. I'm starting to form, in my head, what I want it to be. I like the thought of a collection of short stories, tales about life, what I have been through and where I'm headed. I'm anxious to see how this unfolds – this new project of mine. I want to write about beauty, hope, and fear. I'm not even sure how this differs from journal writing. I guess I just want it to be different somehow, something really special, something others would be interested in reading – something worth writing because this is not just my own therapy, but my gift to the world and especially to my family and friends.

I want to write about beauty, hope, and fear. I'm not even sure how this differs from journal writing. I guess I just want it to be different somehow, something really special, something others would be interested in reading – something worth writing because this is not just my own therapy, but my gift to the world and especially to my family and friends.

I don't think I'll talk about it to anyone. I don't want to be asked about it. I don't want any expectations in case it never really comes together. For some reason I feel like it's important to me. I don't know where or how to begin. I sincerely hope that this will present me with some goals in life because I'm afraid I'm running out of ideas. I really need this idea to work. I can't go on lying on the couch, day after day, stoned on meds and feeling nothing about nothing. That is a very scary and lonely place to be.

The rain is hard and loud tonight. It sounds wonderful! Rebirth – Review – Revise – Recycle – Redo – Begin again. This is what I am hoping for. This is what I need. Wish me luck!

I know my friends love me, but they have dropped off to some degree. It's actually my fault for I have absolutely no desire to return phone calls because I know I'll have to talk about myself and I'm so sick of doing that! Every phone call and card is focused on the cancer so it's always in my face. I know it's all about love but at times I need a respite from that word. I think the constant reference gives it too much power. I just don't want to talk about it any more.

The rain is hard and loud tonight. It sounds wonderful! Rebirth – Review – Revise – Recycle – Redo – Begin again. This is what I am hoping for. This is what I need.

Wish me luck!

What am I? Who am I? Where am I? Why am I? How am I?

November 7, 1999

Today was Lara's baby shower and everyone had a great time. They all said how great I looked which is really because I have gained weight and finally look better. My stomach is still giving me problems, it feels very heavy, bloated, and my right lower abdomen is getting sorer and sorer everyday. It's very localized and sore to the touch. I'm really scared and it's depressing me.

I just want a few weeks or months of wellness. That's all I ask. I don't know why this is happening now and so quickly. I pray that it will fix itself. I will pray and pray hard that this resolves itself and does not amount to anything. I know I'm difficult to please and always seem to be asking for more in this situation but I just don't feel that I should have gotten this horrible disease in the first place. What did I ever do that was so bad?

November 8, 1999

I'm in a bad place again and my right side is still bothering me. I'm afraid to go to the doctor; afraid of the future; afraid of what I have yet to face.

Life has become a series of 'moments to remember'. I'm lucky I don't have many "I wish I had ...." My life has been pretty great and I'm mostly thankful.

Life has become a series of 'moments to remember'. I'm lucky I don't have many "I wish I had ...." My life has been pretty great and I'm mostly thankful.

I've been having nightmares, sometimes two to three a night. They are always persecutory. I am usually running, being chased, or drowning. I am always fighting for my life. Last night I dreamt I was walking along the 401 highway, alone, with water up to my neck. The water kept rising and I seemed to be looking for an exit or a particular place.

I feel disadvantaged, helpless, but all of which I know I am not. I used to be so strong and positive – now most of the time I just feel five years old, alone and very scared. What a life we live. It can be so rich and full and exciting one minute and completely hopeless the next.

I'm trying so hard to ignore this soreness in my side and no luck so far. I will meditate more on this tonight. I will try to fix it myself – I've done it before. I do forget the power of my mind. Ever since the last surgery my connection to the work I'm doing with Alma has been very difficult for me. I used to believe in it sooooo much – why all the doubts now?

> *Our instructions for life aren't written in a procedure manual but answers from within are always available if you 'listen'. Erin mastered this intuitive channel with her inner voice and it gave her clarity when making decisions. Knowing most of her spiritual cleansing was complete; she stopped the intense Metabolic Program and reduced Healing Touch to simple pain relief. Her journal writing became more sporadic but continued to be an outlet for her soul and communication to her future readers.*
>
> *Even though she had reached a level of enlightenment, her human personality chose to continue living every ounce of life possible in the physical world. As Lara said: "To begin with she was fighting to heal herself but later she was fighting for survival and put all her energy there. It was bittersweet."*

My last surgery ended up with somewhat of an illeostomy but not quite. I have a little stomach of sorts on my left side, above my belly button. I have to wear a flange and bag because this is where all of my waste comes out, with the exception of urine – my bladder still works.

I believe I almost died a few months ago in the weeks following the surgery. Sometimes I think the only reason I'm alive is to see my niece/nephew born.

November 21, 1999

What a weekend – the baby was born at 10:46 pm on November 19th and I was thrilled to be present for his birth but I haven't been able to stop crying since it happened. I don't know what's wrong with me. Instead of feeling like I've gained a nephew, I feel like I've lost a sister. I feel so guilty for feeling this awful. I prayed and prayed to God for so long to let me be here to see this happen and I did and I'm so grateful but now it feels almost anticlimactic.

Words keep playing in my head that "Some people stay sick because of all the attention they get." I have always denied that the attention I have received over the last two years has been important to me but now that that attention is threatened and compromised by this beautiful arrival I question myself. Why am I so sad? Why am I so worried about my relationship with Lara? I am an aunt to a beautiful boy named Matthew and everything is as good as it could be right now but mentally and emotionally I'm very fragile.

This whole experience is reminding me that I can never have a child of my own but I know I dealt with those feelings a long time ago. So what makes me cry so much now?

My heart just aches right now as I write this. My life is so far from what I ever thought it would be. I am sad thinking that I will never be in love again and have my own family. I'm jealous, I'm lonely, and I feel completely outside of myself. Why did this have to happen to me?

November 23, 1999

I just got off the phone with Lara and even our conversations are different. She is a typical new Mom with the "Oh! You should see his face …" and "Oh! He's so cute:" and these statements are interjected between our regular conversations.

I know that I feel jealous and get frustrated and don't understand why.

I may be a little frightened as well. I prayed to God to let me live to see Matthew born and now that I was here for the birth I'm afraid of what the future will bring. What do I pray for now? What is my new timeline? Do I pray to make it to Easter, to my next birthday, to Matthew's first birthday???

I guess this is the part where I fall down – but I seem to be having problems getting back up! There is one thing for sure – whether I am up or down I keep going and going and going.

I wish I could enjoy every day and continue to take life one day at a time and be thankful for what I have and how I am. That is the bottom line – Why can't I just be happy?

I get up – I walk – I fall down

Meanwhile I keep dancing.

I guess this is the part where I fall down – but I seem to be having problems getting back up! There is one thing for sure – whether I am up or down I keep going and going and going.

November 28, 1999

My dream last night had me wake up in a bad mood. Maybe if I change my focus and go for a morning walk with a coffee from Starbucks it would help clear my mind. I don't want to waste a day being cranky, life is too short. It's a nice morning outside. Let's see if I can fix myself – I'll get back to you!

It's all a big game. But it's my life and sometimes I feel like I don't know the rules. It's hard to play a game when you don't know the rules – or actually, play a game when there are NO RULES.

Well I just returned from getting a coffee and going for a walk but it hasn't helped my mood. I have to admit that the birth of Matthew, as wonderful as it is, has given me some problems. I fight with my feelings. I look around and see everyone so happy with this event. I'm emotionally so happy but I stop and say WAIT A MINUTE how can we all be so happy when I'm still sick. This, I know is ridiculous but I need to find a way to reconcile that happiness with my illness. I think that is what is so difficult – I don't know how to.

Well it's now 3:00 pm and I've spent half the day completely stoned on pain killers and the other half pacing up and down the length of my apartment trying to figure out why a little new pain or discomfort has the power to completely run my day. I think my brain is really having a hard time processing the fact that I'm as sick as I am and when the pain comes it reminds me and I go into a complete meltdown.

The fact that I'm continuing to live is completely up to me. I mean, I could just admit myself to Palliative Care and decide that

I have had enough. I don't have to live like this. So why do I? It's so hard day after day with this disease. So why continue? Why go on? I mean that very literally.

Boy, sometimes, many times, I just want this to be over, over now. I'm so tired of fighting – so tired of being sad, scared, angry, frustrated and almost manic some days. The uncertainty is the most difficult. I am going to be here for Christmas 1999 and New Years of the new millennium, neither of which I thought would happen. But what do I do then – hope for Valentine's Day? Easter? My thirty-fourth Birthday? It's all a big game. But it's my life and sometimes I feel like I don't know the rules. It's hard to play a game when you don't know the rules – or actually, play a game when there are NO RULES.

Well, its 9:45 pm and I'm in bed, drugged on pain killers. So when I wake up in the morning it will be the moment of truth. I can choose to get out of bed with a negative attitude or I can get up with a positive look at the day ahead. It is COMPLETELY 100% my choice. The pain will still be there, the worry will still be there, the quiet desperation will still be there – so what's it going to be – in spite of all that? I'm hoping and praying that I awake fresh and positive looking forward to the day ahead.

November 29, 1999

Today I awoke in a much better mood than yesterday. I did not have any bad dreams last night. I awoke with my side still sore but I tried to remain positive. The thing to do now is learn to ignore it. The problem with the painkiller is that it does not help the discomfort. Basically, for it to work I have to take an amount that puts me to sleep and I don't want to be sleeping my life away.

I really thought that I would beat this disease two years ago when this nightmare began – how things change. Now I don't know what to think. I actually try not to think about it during the day.

I never think about the future, I don't dwell on the past; I live today as happily as I can but I must say it is still getting harder and harder to do.

I see Lara having a baby; Dad's business closing down; Mom getting new carpets, paint, and wallpaper; and I guess it makes me feel like standing up and screaming HEY! HAVE YOU ALL FORGOTTEN ABOUT THIS NIGHTMARE I'M LIVING?

I can't share in your joys, your news, not truly or honestly because I can't feel anything anymore. I try so hard to take part in everyone else's laughs, joys etcetera but I never really feel what the situation calls for. If everyone is really happy I laugh but not really inside. When someone is telling a story, I try to listen and be involved but I'm not really.

Unless the conversation is about me or my illness I just tune out. I miss being able to feel something for other people. I miss being able to share in other's stories and ups and downs. But I really can't any more.

Unless the conversation is about me or my illness I just tune out. I miss being able to feel something for other people. I miss being able to share in other's stories and ups and downs. But I really can't any more.

I seem to have this need to write a lot the last few days. I think I'm writing a lot to see if I can figure out how I feel about things right now. I feel quite numb and I would like to awaken my feelings to enjoy the days, enjoy the Christmas season that's coming and enjoy the fact that I will get to see the next Millennium – a truly historic moment.

We'll see! We'll see

December 17, 1999

Things had been going along amazingly since I last wrote in here. I'd been feeling REALLY well, going for my walks with a Starbucks every morning and feeling at peace with everything. To top it all off, I even had a terrific doctor's appointment earlier this week. Dr. M. believes that the disease has stabilized and that the hormones that I am taking are working! I immediately called everyone and made their day! I felt guardedly happy, always very guarded. I think it was not a complete happiness because no matter how positive the report, I still have to live such a compromised life!

...the only thing that consistently gets me out of the depression and makes me appreciate what I have is to live for today only and give up trying to control the things I don't have control of! Works every time.

Ironically, the day after my doctor s visit, my stomach and intestines began feeling crampy. I had very loud gurgling sounds and things did not feel like they were digesting. I immediately became absolutely terrified that the good times were over, that I was beginning a downward spiral toward death.

My stomach is okay today. Food is digesting and my ostomy is working. I just have a few more growls than before but what does that really mean? I don't know. All I know is that I am so scared. I used to be okay with the thought of dying but this episode caught me so off guard that it shook my whole foundation.

Lara just called. I love her so much. I feel that I have to stay happy and okay for her. She is so important to me. We talked about Matthew – one of my favorite subjects these days! I spent the day babysitting him yesterday. I enjoyed it soooooo much. They might come over tomorrow. That would be nice.

December 22, 1999

It's absolutely nothing to worry about…..It's absolutely nothing to worry about…..It's absolutely nothing to worry about! It's easy to say but so hard to do. I was chopping up chocolate squares for truffles when I felt something in my armpit. Upon further investigation I discovered a lump, or swollen lymph. I freaked out! I started sweating profusely, I even almost fainted. The tears came easily and quickly. The worst possible scenarios filled my mind. I quickly called the doctor and she was able to see me right away. The first thing she said to me was that there was "absolutely nothing to worry about". She said the lump probably is more cancer but it doesn't mean anything. She thinks I've probably had it for a long time and just never noticed it. I guess that's possible. I think I'm okay.

It's absolutely nothing to worry about…..It's absolutely nothing to worry about…..It's absolutely nothing to worry about!

January 1, 2000

When I get really depressed, like last night, the only thing that consistently gets me out of the depression and makes me appreciate what I have is to live for today only and give up trying to control the things I don't have control of! Works every time. I think this may actually be the secret to getting through this night as happily as humanly possible. Actually, it's the secret to getting through any difficult situation.

HAPPY NEW YEAR!

January 5, 2000

SEARCHING, SEARCHING, SEARCHING.........

Why is it so incredibly difficult for me to decide what I want to do with my life? Am I so lazy that writing a book of some sort is actually not going to happen? Where is the PASSION I used to have about helping others who find themselves in my position? I think I will go through my journals and really start getting serious about putting something together. I don't want to die in vain. I want my insight to help people, even just one other person.

I think I will go through my journals and really start getting serious about putting something together. I don't want to die in vain. I want my insight to help people, even just one other person.

A woman I read about that has been fighting ovarian cancer for 15 years says one of the things you have to do to survive is to volunteer once to twice a week. It's good for your heart and soul. I really need to get serious about something and quickly because this watching TV all day is getting very depressing. My soul is screaming for attention and purpose.

January 15, 2000

It's 2:30 am and I feel compelled to write because this night is a perfect example of the quality of life issues that Dr. B. talked about last summer when we were deciding whether or not I should have the third surgery.

Dr. B. had told my parents to 'let me go' at that point, that a third surgery would only diminish my quality of life to a point that I would be better off dead than alive. I can't believe that seven months later I am alive and fairly well – all because we switched to the more aggressive doctor for one last chance.

The flange and bag that been attached to my body since the last surgery are a going concern and are the major thing that affects my quality of life. I try not to let it prevent me from doing too much but it really restricts me a lot.

Ninety percent of the time I am happy with my life but there is that ten percent that wonders if I should have just let myself go last summer. My life is very compromised compared to how it used to be.

Tonight, it took me an hour of standing in the bathroom naked and cold, waiting for my intestines to empty so I could change the flange and go back to bed. It's all exhausting. This is part of my life now that I have to deal with. It's live like this or not be alive. I really do question this option sometimes.

Ninety percent of the time I am happy with my life but there is that ten percent that wonders if I should have just let myself go last summer. My life is very compromised compared to how it used to be.

January 18, 2000

I prayed for help last night to get myself out of the negative mood I was in all weekend. Today was definitely better. The main thing that is still really bothering me is the way I am a slave to painkillers. I now understand addicts who need their drugs.

What a horrible feeling it is. I am decreasing my doses gradually. I kind of feel overmedicated or I think that's what I'm feeling. I don't know, I've never had a drug problem! I just want to get off this stuff but I know the doctors have told me I can't do it too quickly. I think this has a lot to do with my mood or 'low feelings', depression and lack of energy.

I'm still stuck figuring out exactly what format I want this book to be. I'm leaning towards having it be my story. Honest, emotional, real good advice. I think deep down, I feel that is what is needed out there. Each chapter should take the reader chronologically through my story.

I think I am lazy at heart so I always have a hard time working at things. But as of today and according to my prayers and promises, I am consciously working on my attitude. I am back to walking in the mornings, doing some reading, writing and watching less TV. It's a lot to take on and certainly every day will not be great but I am committed to putting in the effort. With prayers and meditation and a little luck, everything will get better and better. It's my gut feeling.

I'll keep you posted.

With respect to my book, I am slow to start. It has taken me this long just to decide to do it so it will certainly take a few days to really get it going. I am, however, writing a lot in my journal, which I really enjoy. I'm still stuck figuring out exactly what format I want this book to be. I'm leaning towards having it be my story. Honest, emotional, real good advice. I think deep down, I feel that is what is needed out there. Each chapter should take the reader chronologically through my story.

Actually, I do like that. See what happens when you just write, write and write? Things come out completely unexpectedly. Hmmm, Letters to Mathew, let's think about that for a minute …

January 21, 2000

My stomach has been a real problem for the last two days. I have been experiencing a lot of pain, drastically speaking. Food does eventually move through but with pain and that has never happened before. I just don't understand why I'm having so much trouble lately. I'm scared that as I live my life, day to day, waiting for the other shoe to drop, that it is dropping.

Whenever I pray for something to happen, it does. I prayed so hard to gain strength back after my last surgery. I really fought with the idea that it might be time to go when I was in the hospital! But I have felt God's hands and arms carry me when I couldn't carry myself.

All I can do is keep my routine going and just see what happens. I have freaked out before for what turned out to be no reason, although this time seems very different. I guess that's why I'm so scared. I'm not ready to go yet. I have so much more to do! So I pray and pray that everything is okay. And, I pray that if this really is my time that I do go as graciously and courageously as I have fought this horrible, horrible disease. BUT – please don't let it be so!

January 22, 2000

This seems like an okay morning so far, so once again, I have no idea what is wrong with me. Maybe all the prayers are working. I'd like to think it's the prayers because I must say all my prayers (within reason) have been answered up to now. Whenever I pray for something to happen, it does. I prayed so hard to gain strength back after my last surgery. I really fought with the idea that it might be time to go when I was in the hospital! But I have felt God's hands and arms carry me when I couldn't carry myself. I prayed and prayed that I would be here to see Matthew born and I was. I thank God every day for allowing me to know Matthew. He has been an absolute gift.

Thank you God for this chance. All I feel now is so lucky for everything!

Well, so far, my stomach is working beautifully today. I just don't understand what is happening. Maybe I have to stick to soft foods now, or for a while. It's all I can do not to get so nervous when the smallest thing goes wrong. I'm not fooling myself into thinking that everything is all back to normal. I'll believe it when I see it. That's all part of the 'one day at a time' philosophy.

God please bless and help me to cope!

January 23, 2000

This is an emotional roller coaster. I haven't been seeing or calling my friends. Sometimes it's because I'm having a hard time with pain and other times because I'm jealous of what they are doing that I can't. I do get invited out a lot but I never go. If I get lonely I go to Lara's. That is the extent of my social life right now.

January 28, 2000

It's 1:00 am and this is not a good night for sleep. I just woke up again and was having a bit of trouble with my right bag not draining properly and was a little frustrated at having to start another one. All of a sudden, I flashed back to my third surgery and the weeks in the hospital afterward. There was a time when I had nine tubes coming out of me! Nine! I can't believe that I actually came back from all that! I had tubes everywhere! And slowly, one by one they all came out and here I am today, walking around, eating, living – Thank you God for this chance. All I feel now is so lucky for everything!

July 17, 2000

It has been sooooo long since I wrote in this journal and how things have changed. February brought more stomach blockages. February 9th to be exact and into the hospital I went for three weeks. I now have a stomach tube in, that will definitely never come out! It has been a source of help and hurt on different occasions. They perforated a bowel on the way in so I have dealt with various problems from that since it went in. That may have been what caused the tremendous pain after it went in.

Dad says he literally almost put me out of my misery because I was in so much pain after the procedure. The doctors think it was gas that was trapped in my stomach – who knows! Nobody knows anything it seems. I am a big question mark to everyone.

I just returned from another three-week hospital stay. The stomach tube began 'gushing' what turned out to be bowel product to the point where I was literally chained to the couch because of the leaking. They tightened the tube which has helped somewhat with the gushing but not completely.

I feel very confused most of the time. I really don't want to do this anymore. The things I used to find joy in I don't anymore. I'm really miserable. I have just run out of steam. I don't have the energy any more to deal with all this.

July 20, 2000

Well, the verdict is in. There is definitely something wrong with the placement of this tube. Once again, just when things feel like I might be able to get a little peace with all this SHIT – something has to go wrong. I just don't know what to do any more. I am VERY SERIOUSLY on the verge of calling it quits and I think this is the most serious I have been about it. I really just want to die. How do I do that now? I could, tonight, just OD on painkiller, that would do it. Should I? Should/could I really? I have enough of it here and I'm really not joking – let me think – NOW. I think if I just took enough I would just fall asleep.

July 22, 2000

I can't believe I'm actually in the hospital again! My stomach tube has popped into No Man's Land – out of my stomach and it seems it is no longer useful. My worst nightmare has come true in that they may have to put in another tube. How can this be happening to me? Right now I feel No God, No Jesus, helping me. I am alone despite what the scriptures say. It is not true. I really think I'm being called back and this is how it happens. By getting rid of my options and leaving me with slow starvation. Isn't that nice? All I do is sit here and shake my head that this is even happening because I really can't believe it. It is the ONE THING I prayed for not to happen and it does.

I'm sick to death of seeing all these things as 'challenges' in life. How many 'challenges' do I have to endure before saying enough is enough and just letting go?

July 28, 2000

Well, speaking of challenges, I'm back in the hospital AGAIN with an abscess in my stomach. There is a fluid collection around my old colostomy and scar that is going to have to be lanced tomorrow morning to let all the fluid out. Although I'm very grateful that that is all it turned out to be I find myself once again, feeling very sorry for myself.

July 29, 2000

I have pain this morning. My abscess is really sore. I hope the lancing helps. It is such a beautiful day outside I should be out there with my friends! God I'm depressed. I am living in this blue funk, in pain wondering how much is enough? I wanted life so much but for some reason it is not mine to have. I wish so hard. I wish until I cry. I don't know what more I can do! It's very lonely in here.

This is without a doubt the worst mental day I have ever had. I am in the darkest place I have ever been in. It is awful! I have put a NO VISITORS sign on the door and unplugged the phone. I have agreed to stay in the hospital until I feel safe.

> *I arrived at the hospital and Erin wouldn't let anyone in her room. It was a big blow for me, like a door slamming in my face. I knew I shouldn't take it personally – it was something she was going through. Still it was painful, and I realized why therapists and doctors stay somewhat distant from patients, so they don't get hurt.*

August 6, 2000

It's early morning and I'm actually in Victoria at Dad and Sylvia's debating whether or not to get up! I made it over yesterday feeling semi-human! I, along with the nurses and doctors, felt that I should get out of the hospital for a while. It's going okay so far – but I'm not out of bed yet!

August 8, 2000

I'm back from Victoria and in the hospital. I am going home tomorrow. I'm a little nervous about going home so quickly but yesterday and today have both been uneventful and relatively smooth. I will just go home and take it as it comes.

August 9, 2000

If only all my days could be mornings. I feel so good in the morning – normal. I'm lying here in bed debating whether or not to go for walk while enjoying a brownie before breakfast. I think I slept well. I know I slept well!

August 15, 2000

Dad and I had a terrific meeting with Dr. M. yesterday. I feel really good about the information she gave us about my choosing to call it quits whenever I want to. It won't be terribly painful. She figures my problem will probably stem from dehydration in which case my kidneys and liver will stop working. I would remain very sedated and probably become somewhat confused because of the chemical imbalance in my body. I would virtually become weak and comatose and just pass.

I feel really good about the information she gave us about my choosing to call it quits whenever I want to.

August 19, 2000

How can everything go from relative comfort to absolute suffering all in twelve hours? My mornings are still pretty good and yet by 1:00 pm things start going downhill until I'm miserable by bedtime.

I feel my time is drawing near. It's not even hard to admit. It's actually almost a comfort to look forward to no more suffering. I would just miss everyone so much. I don't know how to say goodbye. I feel like there are still a lot of loose ends to tie up – letter to Matthew, a bit of a will and letters to some people etcetera.

Letter to Mathew

Little Peanut,

This is both the easiest and hardest letter for me to write. It's easiest because it is to you and there is so much I'd like to tell you. It's hardest because the reason I wanted to write to you is because I won't be able to enjoy the incredible privilege and joy of watching you grow up. I want you to know first and most importantly to me that to have been able to see you being born and grow in your first year of life has been the greatest joy of my life. You are the most precious little person I have ever known. Unfortunately and for reasons that can never be known, I got a very bad disease called cancer and it will cause me to die just before your first birthday. It's a complicated sickness and one that is very unfair so I won't go into a lot of details about it but maybe your Mom can explain it to you when you are old enough to understand. For now, I just wanted to share a few things with you that I wish I could do in person.

You have to know, first of all, that you have been born into a very special family. You will always be safe and secure and so loved and have everything you need.

That is a promise I know I can make to you. Your Mom and Dad will always be honest with you and try to make the best decisions for you so remember that even if you don't agree with them all the time they are always thinking of what is in your best interest and what will be best for you. I have a feeling that you are going to be a very strong, stubborn, intelligent person so when disagreements happen with Mom and Dad, remember how much they love you and only want what's best for you.

There is a picture attached to this letter where I am feeding you your bottle and our eyes are very connected. Since the day you were born I have felt this special connection with you. You stare deeply into my eyes and mine into yours and I feel the deepest sense of trust and love. I hope you felt it too.

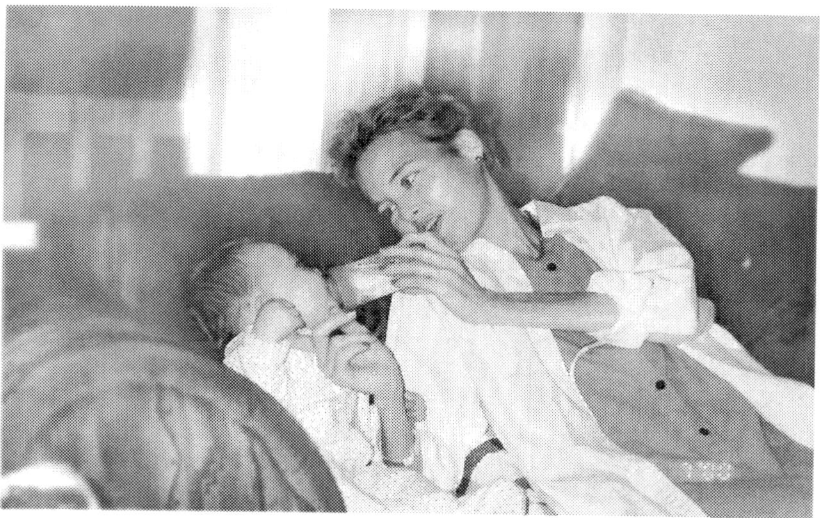

August 21, 2000

It seems that the decision has been made that I would be better off in Palliative Care. Things are getting harder and harder and I am having trouble handling everything. I waiver between going there and staying home but then I think its right. I think it's worth a try. Besides, I don't know how long it would take to get a bed.

Well, I'm going into Palliative Care tomorrow morning! They have a bed for me so soon! I'm very pleased about it. I think it's meant to be. I found another hole in my stomach today!?! Isn't that just a kick in the head? It confirms my need to be in Palliative and also says to me that it's really over. I don't think that everyone realizes this but I will never leave Palliative. I will die there and sooner rather than later. The thing now is how do I begin the process? When is best?

August 23, 2000

I'm in Palliative now and feeling more confused than ever. I don't know when to start my impending demise. I feel like the decision has to be made but I don't know how to make it and no one can tell me when or how. It's all up to me and I'm really confused. Saying 'Go' is really scary only in that I worry for my family – and it's so final. Maybe I can hang on a little longer. Maybe I could go to the cottage on Pender with Lara. I don't know. I don't know. Actually I could not go to the cottage. As much as I think I could, I know it won't happen.

I don't know when to start my impending demise. I feel like the decision has to be made but I don't know how to make it and no one can tell me when or how. It's all up to me and I'm really confused.

I really feel like I want this to be over but I'm afraid to end it. I'm afraid to set the wheels in motion. I wish it would just happen. That I wouldn't have to decide – it would be so much easier. I feel so guilty about the timing of everything. Everyone is so busy right now.

August 24, 2000

I'm eating less and less and becoming more and more tired. This is something I can control because I just get so sick of eating and then dealing with all the leaking of my tubes. It's easier to just not eat. I know that if I don't start eating I will get more and more tired and eventually just sleep all the time.

August 25, 2000

Dad's coming in tonight. I'm really looking forward to seeing him. I'm counting on him to put my 'end' into play. I really think I'll start this weekend to seriously stop eating. I need his support to do this. For some reason I need his support more than anyone else's. I feel like he's the one with the power to 'let me' let go. I'm so ready – I just don't know how to.

When we talk to Dr. M., I want to tell her that I'm ready to go. Oh God, please help me to do that! I feel so ready – it's exciting to think of never having to change another tube or dressing, never worrying about how much I eat, going to a place, although unknown, that is nothing but happy and positive and lovely.

But Oh God please don't make me wait long. I'm a little afraid of that I must admit. I wish I had no choice and it just started. Making 'the call' is really terrifying. It's so final. But that's what I want. My writing gets so small because I keep falling asleep-------
----

This is Erin's last journal entry.

In her last few months, Erin slipped in and out of consciousness with a plea to her mother "Mom, I just want my life back," then final acceptance, as her last words to her father were: "Dad, will you read me the Bible?"

Memorial Notice

HIGGINS – Erin Leigh Ann passed away on Tuesday, October 17, 2000, age 34 years, after a very brave and courageous battle with ovarian cancer.

Erin passionately loved her family and friends; how blessed we were to have had her in our own lives! She taught us all about bearing great adversity with even greater courage and dignity:

God saw you were getting tired
When a cure was not to be
So He closed His arms around you
And whispered "come to me"
You didn't deserve what you went through
And so He gave you rest
God's garden must be beautiful
He only takes the best.
So when we saw you sleeping
So peaceful and free from pain
We could not wish you back
To suffer that again

"Spirituality is always there. It's when you make friends with it (your soul) that you become who you truly are."

Epilogue

I believe from somewhere within, Erin had chosen to experience a full lifetime in just a few years. It created a snowball effect for rapid inner growth and had exponential results. All of us around her were caught up in this dynamic experience through a whirlwind of unstoppable events.

Her last year was a question mark for many but Erin didn't like missing anything and wanted to live that last piece of life. The only reason her body survived as long as it did is because – she was Erin – only willing to leave on her own terms and when she was totally ready. Her earthly mission was not yet complete for her even thought the daily difficulties and humiliation to do with physical wear and tear plagued her. She was no longer her old self and these limitations took a toll on her spirit - but to keep on keeping on was heroic.

People took the time out of their busy schedules just to 'be' with Erin. Those times with her were intimate in many ways – from working with tubes that ran her body to helping her shower and dress. Her friend Kathy told me she felt privileged to be part of that intimacy but more so, was the time spent talking at a soul level about genuine deep feelings. This final bonding time offered spiritual growth for everyone including friends and friends of friends that formed an extended circle around Erin's journey.

Erin left no stones unturned and nothing unfinished. When she chose to complete her journey we knew she left in peace and a legacy of inspiration and teachings for others.

PART II

Other Stories:

By Alma Lightbody

"Life and Death are but different phases of Being.
You are part of the eternal Life"
~ Paramahansa Yogananda

CHAPTER 7

Pieces of the Puzzle

"Life is like a game, you can't win them all and yet the game goes on, forcing all to play."

In my relationship with Erin, which was on many levels, I got to know her very well and was truly impressed with her strength and courage in the face of such adversity. Initially, Erin came for energy treatments almost weekly and our discussions were usually deep and serious but through the layers there was always humour and fun.

Erin was adamant about researching her dis-ease and with that wanted to share all that she was learning with others. Her journals were a major resource for her to expound her feelings as well as to document her findings with an ongoing desire to use them to write a book and share her story. She wanted to help others 'heal' themselves. In the last year the difference between 'healing the soul' and 'curing the body' came into conflict for her. She had been sure she would achieve both. Even though the curing evaded her and she began to question her purpose, she never lost her passion to write a book about her journey.

One of her last wishes was that her journals be passed on to me to compile her book. With that invitation, two years later I met with the challenge to fulfill Erin's wish to use her journals and share her experiences, insights and advice.

While collecting information, by reading her journals and interviewing friends and relatives, I sensed there was a force, greater than I understood, in the Universe. Something appeared to be blocking the progress of the project. Information did not come to me readily. Interviews were postponed and one key piece of valuable information – the video about Erin – produced by a friend for a journalling course, was missing. In fact the original plus the only copy seemed to have disappeared.

A wonderful true story that touched many of us was obtaining permission from Erin, two years after her passing, to use her journals to tell her story.

Coincidentally, at the same time a rather innocent event about a puzzle took place with Lara's son, Matthew. A special wooden toy puzzle he cherished was missing some pieces and he was frantic. Lara searched the house from stem to stern with no luck. The missing pieces could not be found. Somehow, this seemed to us to relate back to when Erin was diagnosed with cancer, and she began to reconstruct the pieces of her personal puzzle as she began her unknown journey.

I needed some help here and asked Lara if she'd ever had any spiritual contact with Erin since her passing. Lara told me that Erin visited her routinely, sometimes very clearly and other times it was just a knowingness. At one time Lara had prayed and asked Erin for help with an issue she was dealing with and Erin was there and they laughed and cried together. She then told me, the last time Erin visited was quite a while ago. "Sometimes it might be just a breath on my hand but I know it's her."

I asked Lara if she was willing to try and contact Erin to help us through this stalemate. The question was: did Erin want this book produced?

Finally, with some trepidation, Lara was able to create a space that worked for her – a quiet place, a picture of Erin, along with Erin's favorite music and the intent to make contact with her. Without spoken words or a great vision, Lara was confident she connected with and felt Erin's presence so put forth the question about whether she wanted the book to be created.

The next morning Lara's father called to say he had found the 'missing video' and right after the phone call her son came out of his room and said "Mommy, I found the pieces to the puzzle."

Clearly, it seemed the story of the lost items and the found items was an encoded message from Erin that it was okay to proceed with the book.

Following these events two more timely things happened. An interview I had been trying to set up for many months with Erin's closest friends happened the day after the video and the pieces of the puzzle were found. Then Lara told me that her family had just spent time at Erin's memorial site to honour the second anniversary of her passing. It seemed to Lara that "Everything was okay with Erin now."

Things were now falling easily into place. The final piece of this story was a channeled message, via automatic writing, from Erin during one of my meditations a month later. It was her bridge between life and death. The message follows, written in first person as received.

> "Alma, I found the pieces of the puzzle – it was about my heart. It was finding the pieces that were missing, damaged, broken and empty. Pieces I had given away to others and never retrieved. Some of this life journey had picked away at my sense of being. I know part of it was my life's plan from previous lives but nevertheless it was in my face this time.
>
> It's amazing how bit by bit we give away pieces of ourselves to others and don't even think about or

consider trying to get those pieces back. It's all so much clearer to me now that I can look at the overall picture from a much higher perspective. It's a time for me of reviewing how I made out in that recent incarnation. I look at what cards were dealt and how I played the game. My parent's divorce broke my heart and for a while I lost some of their pieces of my puzzle. With my own marriage, I needed to learn how I was losing my own identity and understand when to walk away.

But, you know during my illness, best time–worst time, all of these missing pieces plus extra came back to me in such a profound way. It was something I would never have imagined. The love I was looking for to fill my empty heart was right there all the time and the love and support of friends, family, support workers and people I didn't even know brought back all the pieces of my heart. The deep unconditional love was so powerful it pieced my heart and soul back together.

If I had not been physically ill I would have worked, had a family, coached soccer, played with my pets but in actuality I may have never found that 'wholeness of being' that I achieved in that short bout with cancer. Through that dis-ease my emptiness of heart was filled ten-fold by the power of love around me.

The close, intimate times and discussions with those close to me only happened because of the physical illness that pushed me to that point of remembering what my soul really needed for its true fulfillment. The cancer also brought forth a purpose from within to teach and help others.

In my last few months I became cranky and a little angry with friends that were able to go on living. I wasn't able to comprehend the whole picture clearly from the drugged state I lived in. I was also unhappy with you because the energy work hadn't healed my body. That was also part of my journey I so badly needed to understand. "Healing is about the soul and doesn't always include the body."

The love from the earthly plane is still powerful but in a new way for me now. I can understand how the physical form and the controls society places on it, is hampered by a tunnel vision that makes it difficult for the soul to make its presence known, but from my present perspective it's now so clear.

There is another part of truth I need to share with you. Looking at things from the above mentioned perspective didn't come immediately or easily. When I left the physical plain, I was still "pissed off" at being short-changed in a life that I felt was finally taking off for me. I was exactly where I wanted to be; back in Vancouver with family and friends and in a job that was something I had dreamed of, so why me??

At the end, I became disillusioned and was no longer sure about what to say in my book because initially it was supposed to be about teaching people how to get well and survive cancer. When you began to talk to my family about this book I was not receptive to the idea so was 'not available' to contact but then a series of things happened that helped change my mind.

My family and friends gathered on my birthday two years after I had left the physical plain. The ceremony was simple but the love in that circle was so profound and genuine that it continued to fill my soul. Then, my direct blood family spent the anniversary of my passing at the memorial site with me. It was like old times with everyone chatting and connecting and Dad even smoked a cigar, just like the old days. Those pieces of the broken puzzle had reformed in a different way and there was a wholeness to it that helped me feel my earthly mission was now complete.

Alma, I know you sensed a block from me about compiling the book and asked Lara to contact me to ask if I wanted the book to be written. This was tough because I had shut the idea down and now I had to make a decision but you know it was not that hard. The previous happenings had helped me to feel complete so once again I was ready to share my story. Throughout my journey it had been my desire and purpose so how could I ignore it now?

My next challenge was about how to pass on my message of acceptance and yes, there was excitement about the manifestation of my dream to teach others. With a little slight of hand, the lost tapes were easy to make 'available' and my wonderful nephew was a receptive conduit to complete my message with "Mom, I found the pieces to the puzzle."

All pieces of my heart and soul are back together in a wonderful new wholeness filled with unconditional love. I am at peace and may the words from my journals help others find wholeness and peace as well.

Au Revoir, Erin xxoo

CHAPTER 8

Insights

"People come into your life for a reason, a season or a lifetime."

The first portion of this book was a visit through Erin's journals as she spoke from the depth of her soul and exposed her inner most feelings and emotions. It was the deep side of her psyche, a place that most people never connect with themselves. It was like the back or darker side of a mirror.

The insights shared by family and friends in this section are like the front of the mirror and reflect how they saw the bright side that portrays her vibrant personality, courage and strength that others admired and learned from.

The interviews in this section are the exact wording of family and friends. They talk about what a legacy Erin left and how profoundly each of their lives were changed as they shared her journey. Her courageous story wove itself through many layers of friends and family and left an imprint on each of us.

<u>Alma:</u> "Erin didn't realize the gift she gave me when she left me her journals to share with others. Compiling this work has been a profound experience I will hold in my heart forever."

<u>Kathy and Jen</u>

These girls had a very strong ten-year bond and were all powerful people. Kathy flew home from Taiwan, where she was working, on a couple of occasions just to 'be' with Erin. Jen is a singer that worked in local clubs and so was more available to spend time with Erin. They were all very close.

This interview was with the two of them together so their words are intermingled.

"People that were around us and didn't even know Erin as intimately as we did wanted to understand and learn and be part of the bigger lesson, the bigger picture, and not in a voyeuristic way. To look back now at the experience, it was an honour and privilege to be that close to it all.

Erin was always a teacher. She taught by telling stories and it was how she told them – pragmatic and logical. She gave them a sense of realism. She talked about her own experiences as she proceeded through her journey. She was passionate about reading and learning things about herself, her illness and her diet.

In her determination, she read the newspaper every day to keep up to date. We wouldn't have done that but it was her way of keeping in control and in touch. She talked about politics and the highlights of what was going on. We couldn't believe it. We never saw her so involved before. Then she helped her step-sister find an apartment when she moved to Vancouver. Erin would look through the paper and from her hospital bed she would phone and ask questions then leave her hospital number for people to call her back – so incredible!

Erin put everyone else first. She looked after her siblings, was a referee for her parents and motherly to her husband but she didn't take care of herself. I'll never forget when Erin came back to Vancouver after her divorce.

It was at a hockey gig – she wore jeans and a red turtle neck sweater. I said 'You look awesome.' She answered, 'Maybe on the outside but on the inside my self esteem is pretty low.' She internalized everything – she was a classic case of 'everything is fine'. We never knew anything was wrong with her marriage.

On her video Erin said 'Knowing what I know today, I don't think I would change anything.' I can't comprehend how she felt but isn't it sad that we have to get sick in order to know how much people care about us?

Even before she was diagnosed she just loved to live. Some people love to live but Erin really loved to live! She played hard and worked hard and enjoyed people.

I think Erin was optimistic at the beginning, we all were. It wasn't until the third surgery where she almost died – we were all on pins and needles for weeks and then she survived. We finally realized she was terminal. Towards the end Erin didn't do everyday things anymore. She just wanted to talk about where she was going. We really had to be up for those conversations – some people couldn't do that. You are together a lot and what you do is talk. Her family and friends were with her all the time 24-7."

Jen: "I was able to share these feelings with Erin as I sat by her bed. Sometimes she'd say she was ready to go and closer to the end she'd say this isn't fair, this isn't right and 'why me?' I didn't know how to answer that.

What I can say is from the diagnosis through the whole journey I was totally in awe of her strength and her doggedness. She was completely focused. I was so amazed at her drive and vision and I know it's affected my life.

I was able to make decisions about past and current relationships because of Erin. I realize life is too short. I somehow learned, through her pain and agony. Today whenever I'm lost I say what would Erin do now? Her advice was always sound – with or without cancer. Her advice was clear. Why are you wasting your time on that or what's holding you back? Just do it."

Kathy: "We helped her shower and bathe – things we wouldn't ordinarily do. It touches you very deeply. I had this incredible and moving experience – only a few of us were close enough to her to hear her crying – it was most impactful. Also in the intimacy of cleaning her tubes – she allowed me into her body. I am spiritual and really understand that our body is just a vessel and hers was a beautiful vessel. I loved talking to it and hearing her laugh. I love that laugh.

At the end, as well as close friends and family, people that knew Erin from previous jobs, extended circles of friends, people that didn't even know her wanted to, or did come to her funeral. The Church was packed. Relatives traveled from all across Canada."

Christine

"From the time we first met, where we worked at the Waterfront Hotel, we clicked right away. Erin embodied strength and a stubbornness that was very appealing because I loved a good argument and an assured response. Our relationship developed seeing eye-to-eye on a lot of issues as well as becoming partners in crime. What I mean is we were definitely a team when it came to dancing and partying. I found it refreshing to know someone who wasn't afraid to tell me exactly how she felt. She was a good listener and had a radiating smile that sent warmth throughout any room.

Erin's strength was taking care of others, always being there for her friends and family but I rarely saw Erin take the time to take care of herself. I don't believe Erin wanted to leave Vancouver to go back to Toronto but she did it for her husband. He was very dominant but good at making it seem like he was open-minded. She rarely talked about their problems but since I was sometimes present it was difficult not to stick my nose in. To what capacity do you leave a good friend in a potentially harmful situation? Was I meddling?

A few years later, with an unfriendly divorce in process Erin returned to Vancouver with a huge emotional burden as well as the need to find a job. That is a lot for anyone to handle.

My reaction to Erin's diagnosis was initially shock. I will never forget the doctor's own reactions. I believe it was the most difficult news he had had to deliver and considered walking right past the room where her family and friends were waiting. Doreen, being a nurse, was the one that kept composed and asked a lot of questions. I remember thinking how lucky Erin was to have such a wonderful mom. She was the strength in that room.

Throughout the first months I maintained that Erin was going to get through this. Why wouldn't she? She was determined and strong, surrounded by a loving and supportive family and friends as well as a good team of doctor's.

I thought a lot about what I knew of Erin's life and am convinced that this could have been prevented. Everyone has the potential to get cancer. It is aggravated by stress, pollution, eating habits and poor emotional, physical and mental habits. The last three are big ones because as humans we don't pay attention to the fact that our daily thoughts and habits can quickly manifest into an unhealthy physical state."

Kim

"At the hospital, after we found out it was cancer I broke down in tears. Erin grabbed my hand and said "We're going to fight this." I believed her. She seemed incredibly strong from the very beginning. My mom had survived ovarian cancer and so could Erin.

It reaffirmed that we all have challenges to face and I believe things happen for a reason. It's too bad when we have to learn from someone else's misfortune but I wouldn't change having shared part of Erin's journey. It makes you look at little things differently and appreciate them so much more.

Physically, the changes in Erin seemed slow – short hair, then no hair and then she began to wear wigs and hats. I remember one time I went to Monk McQueen's to see her and didn't even recognize her. She wore a black bobbed wig and looked fantastic. I got the feeling she felt that way too – just the way she carried herself.

On one of the best days of my life, I shared the whole day with Erin. I met her at Solly's who makes the best cinnamon buns in the Lower Mainland. Unfortunately she couldn't have any because of her bowel problems but she just liked to come out.

We spent the rest of the day running errands and having fun.

That night we went to see Jen sing in a new band and there I met my husband. I vividly remember that day and how the sun shone, spending a good quality day with Erin – the world just felt right.

Near the end there were huge, drastic changes to her body and when we went for a walk everyone was looking at her. Erin just seemed to take it in stride, as she always did.

I always felt comfortable asking Erin questions about what was going on. Sometimes she didn't want to see anyone and that was understandable but difficult because I wanted to be helpful. When I sat with her alone that last time I believe she could hear us. I told her it was okay to let go. We would miss her but she needed to stop fighting and have a rest. She was going to a good place and I know she believed that.

Even now it is still helpful for me when I hear from her family because there was an incredible bond created for all of us sharing Erin's journey."

Phillipa

Phillipa, not available for an interview, is a manager at Monk McQueen's Restaurant where Erin worked as Sales Manager. They became good friends and Phillipa provided excellent support for Erin as she balanced her chemo treatments and surgeries with work.

Working and being motivated was extremely important for Erin and the support she received from all the staff was amazing. She blossomed when setting up and managing parties and functions.

"You were a good hire when I hired you and you're still my best hire"

Sean, Erin's Brother

"Her diagnosis was a tough moment for sure, probably the toughest in my life. We were genetically alike so I also felt threatened. My fears were mostly for her but it took me sometime to deal with the possibility of my own mortality. I almost felt guilty at times. It kind of gave me a zest for life and I learned to appreciate the moment.

Where did all her courage come from? Erin didn't show the dark moments.

She was very independent and remained open to possibilities. She knew it was a struggle for everyone around her. She wasn't selfish, she listened to others, but she must have felt alone with that kind of challenge.

I often wondered how it could have been prevented, avoided, but there are no excuses. It's a waste of time to wonder why. There's no blame in the end – it's an unfair thing. You can do all the things to help prevent it but in the end it can happen to anyone – no fault, no blame, and no justification.

Terminal illness sends the person and everyone around them through purgatory. I guess it would be nice to just hold onto what's important and not dig into things too deeply. At some time we have to accept what is extremely complex. It's good to be grateful for what you have.

I believe much more in soul now. I have faith in an after life now. It's comforting. In a way it was a most challenging and enriching time. Severe challenges push us deeper to look for answers."

Lara, Erin's Sister:

"When I learned about her diagnosis everything felt spaced out and unreal. For a week I cried uncontrollably and was unable to move. Everything was dark and it was never going to get light again – like I was in a slowed down spaced out world. Things seemed to take forever – even walking by a house.

Erin didn't change how strong she lived until she died. She liked to talk about life. She touched people so much and they just wanted to be around her. Helping others gave her stability and control.

She always asked other people what was happening with them and loved to tell stories about what she was learning. She was a pillar for her friends, direct and helpful right to the end. We are all here to learn and some lessons are harder than others. For Erin, cancer was a vehicle for her to teach others. She changed everyone around her.

Spiritually, there was growth – her skin was glowing. She was radiant from within and began to find out who she was. I hadn't seen her look so beautiful. She was meditating, eating well, journal writing and taking care of her own healing.

When she was married it was all about her husband and she didn't know who she was. During her illness she had some 'me' time to find out who she was. I think everyone should take the time to do that.

At times the subject of the 'missing the babies' she couldn't have came up but she didn't dwell on it or feel sorry for herself. In her heart she had always wanted a house with a white picket fence, a husband, kids and dogs but today was a new day.

Erin loved partying, dancing and dinner parties. Even when she was in complete survival mode she would plan parties and make sure her makeup was just right before attending. On my birthday, Erin got off the couch in front of the TV and got all dolled up and took a cab to my office with a birthday cake. She loved things like that. What was powerful was just being with her.

Healing Touch had been able to help her and calm her down but at the end she didn't want to do that anymore. She had become disillusioned and disappointed she hadn't been healed. That work did help her. I put a lot of value on it.

To begin with, she was fighting to heal herself but later she was fighting for survival and put all her energy there. She didn't even want to see her friends at the end because they could do things that she couldn't – it was bitter sweet. She had a hard time letting go. I knew from the day she was diagnosed she would go 'kicking and screaming;' she didn't want to give up.

This whole experience totally changed my life. I was materialistic, worked at a brokerage house and it was all about money. I learned if I had a million dollars I'd still be heart broken. After Erin's death we moved to a simpler life and cut living expenses by forty thousand dollars a year. I go to local markets and ride my bicycle to work. We don't have cable TV or internet. I try to cook more, we go for hikes and I spend more time on my relationship with Steve. I owe all that to Erin. The quality of life is so much better and there is such a value in family and community. I speak about Erin to other people and it makes a difference. It brings people back to earth. It's hard to go against the grain regarding hair, nails and body-beautiful but I now have a better awareness about what's really important."

Doreen, Erin's Mom

"Things moved along very quickly from the MRI to the surgery and I was 80% sure the results wouldn't be good. Because of her attitude and strength I was hopeful it could be contained for a while. I felt upset for her because she had just started her dream job and had been through so much with her divorce in the last while. Being a nurse, I knew she was going to need all the stamina she could come up with. It would have been easier if it was me.

Erin didn't show much emotion. She was rational, clinical and stoic and wanted to know everything in detail – what is happening? – what are the results? – then she accepted them and went on to the next step. The only time she really lost it with a panic attack was when she woke from surgery and found she had a colostomy bag. She thought the bag meant they had got the cancer because that had been the deal but the doctors told her it didn't work as expected.

Even though she was loving to all and outgoing there was part of her that was almost resentful about her adversity in life. She was a caretaker with family and relationships and never had a chance to work on herself. She was upset about our divorce. The one point that I would make is that Brian and I wrongly didn't involve the kids in our decisions. I don't think that was fair. They had no chance to express how they felt or have a chance for input.

Erin was strong, persistent and showed strength of character – making decisions whether right or wrong. These attributes really came through when she was ill. She wanted to make her own decisions without unsolicited advice on a daily basis. She included family for major decisions but didn't want us to interfere and that's fair.

Erin made lists and checked them off till she died. She was Erin till she died. She was even stubborn about taking too many painkillers. She didn't want to become addicted. She often refused to try different drugs if she didn't know enough about them. Near the end in Palliative Care Erin said to me 'Mom I just want my life back, I have an ache in my heart.' She knew she wasn't going to make it but never accepted it, not for a second. Control was a big issue with everything.

This experience changed my life profoundly and it hasn't been the same since. I could never have perceived any of my children dying before me. Many priorities change but life goes on, it doesn't stand still. I still go to work and do what I need to do but losing Erin affects every day.

I try to live more in the moment. My advice is to enjoy your children, have fun with them and don't get bogged down in the small stuff."

Brian, Erin's Dad

(From a card) "If you hadn't been 'chemo-ing' today I might not have stopped to think of how special you are and always have been to me. Here's to love and life, my little tiger, Love Dad

How to find more of herself with each passing day was a strength of Erin's. It's hard to know where she found that strength continually. In day to day life we are not usually challenged to the 'nth' degree. We are unaware of the hidden resources we can tap into. She found them. Erin maintained a wholeness of life and found ways to enjoy it – never willing to throw in the towel. She went back to work right after surgery. She needed purpose and loved her work.

I spent more time with Erin in those last few years than I would have if she had lived till she was eighty. It made me older and wiser. It was the real stuff of life, the real truth, the bare bones..

She touched some great highs in the lives of everyone around her. Wondrous things and funny things came out at times. One morning at 2:00 am she needed help and said 'Dad could you reach me that syringe?' She was giving herself an injection, with tubes all around her and said 'Dad, I'm glad I'm not a paraplegic – that would be real hard to handle.'

The Ultimate Moment of absolute poignancy was at Erin's place near the end. She had a gushing wound on her belly and her tubes were leaking. I took her into the shower, my 34-year-old daughter just skin and bones.

It's amazing when you see a body that emaciated and coming apart yet the spirit was still strong. I've never been faced with such a juxtaposed position. The spirit was something other than her body. The body is only a vehicle. It was an illumination for me that our body is not us – she was something other than her body. It was going to wrack and ruin. I had always thought the body housed the spirit but my sister's vision was that spirit was a big presence hobbled by the body.

Erin's last words were, 'Dad, will you read me the Bible?' Three days later when she passed she had clearly left her body. It was a celebration, I was euphoric – she was at peace."

"Only when you drink from the river of silence shall
You indeed sing
And when you have reached the mountain top, then
You shall begin to climb.
And when the earth shall claim your limbs, then
you shall truly dance."
~ Kahlil Gibran

Afterword

Erin's father called me at 5:00 am on October 17, 2000 to tell me Erin had passed on. After some quiet meditation I sat down with relief and sadness and wrote Erin this letter:

Dear Erin,

Love is something that's hard to put a value on. It's so profound and deep but something we can't touch in our literal and material world. Yet you taught us how to transcend that barrier and took us deeper into our feelings and our hearts than we ever thought possible.

It wasn't a planned lesson by far, but one that just evolved with each moment of our experience with and through you, as you dealt with your journey with cancer.

In our own way we all experienced the classic stages of loss and death: Denial, Anger, Negotiation, Depression and finally Acceptance. We dealt with it at different times and in different ways, while you 'the captain of our team' continued to forge ahead, beating the odds at each turn in the road.

It took you a long time to consider the stage of 'acceptance' as an option. I remember our talk near the end of your life on earth. You said to me, "You know, I was always sure I could beat this – I didn't believe I was going to die." We talked then about how it's not always the physical body that is healed in the process of 'healing' but it may serve as a vehicle for spiritual healing and transcendence to wholeness of mind, body and soul.

We know that you, as our leader and captain achieved this spiritual goal and in the process we all reached a new level of growth and enlightenment we hadn't planned for, but will carry with us forever.

Erin, thank you for the opportunity to work with you and for the love we'll always share.

This morning our souls connected during my meditation and you gave me permission to disconnect your energetic centres from your physical body. It was a wonderful experience to help you move into a higher realm. I know it was hard for you to 'let go'. You always wanted to be in control and letting go was not easy for you. Now that you have left the earth plain, I know you are aware of how beautiful the spirit world is with it's ambience of light, peace and harmony.

Today I'm very sad from a human standpoint and I know that's okay. Grieving is natural and I'll really miss you. I'm burning a candle for you to help your passage and the picture of us together last Christmas sits on the table beside it. I'm also drinking from the teacup you gave me for the new house on Pender. The house isn't ready yet but I thought it was okay to use the cup today. I know you touched it to wrap it – so I only washed the inside before drinking from it. Thank you.

I'm also babying the small pine tree you gave us last Christmas and it will find a special place at Pender. I remember how much you loved the Island and how our relationship grew as we spent many special times together.

Your life journey had begun to give messages at a deeper, more contemplative level and that's not always an easy place for many of us to go. We're not trained to do so and are often fearful of what we might find there. Us poor humans, we have this fixation about change, fear and death. We think they are awful, so we aren't willing to step into another realm where we might see things from a different perspective or unbelievably look at life's 'whole picture'.

You've gone into that realm now and what a beautiful place that must be without human restrictions from words like *can't, don't,* and *should.* I'm sure you'll have a few chuckles as you watch us earthlings continue with our restricted existence. We don't 'get it' that thoughts-create-reality but you'll see it first hand and it will be instantaneous.

As I look at this picture of you, your eyes are smiling and a dove sits off to the right of your head. There's a wonderful lightness in your face yet underneath the coveralls there are tubes and bags protruding from your fragile body.

You were great at putting on a good face and not letting the cancer project its outward manifestations of 'Here I Am'. You didn't ask for pity or act helpless with 'poor me'. Your independence and strength made it hard for some of us to realize what you were going through. Yet there was warmth at the soul level that grew throughout your journey.

I never had children of my own and you found a place deep in my heart, waiting to hold love for a special person. That love will always be part of me. I believe as I work with people I hold unconditional love for each of them but you took me to new depths and meaning for that love.

The last time we talked and said 'goodbye' it was a very profound experience to be able to speak about death so openly and clearly. We also talked about the book you had wanted to write and would still like to see written. As we've said before, whatever is meant to be will be. You can help with the story from the spirit realm and I'm happy to be your 'medium'.

Love forever – Au Revoir! Alma

Postscript:

Well Erin, ten years later – mission accomplished. Your purpose is fulfilled and your book is complete and ready for printing.

It's yours now to take into the Universe to help others.

With Love, Light & Blessings,

Alma

About the Authors

Erin Higgins

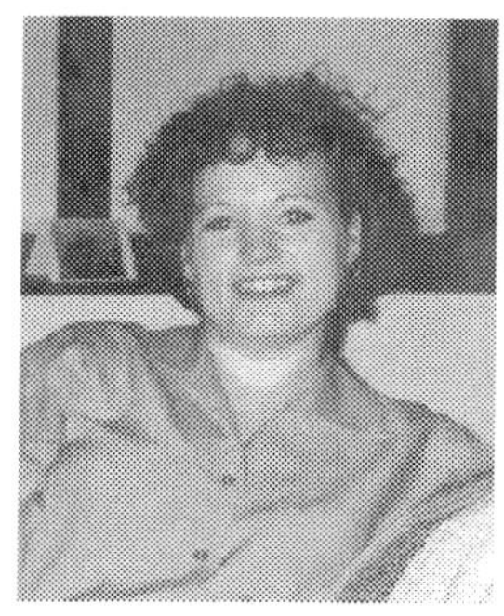

The eldest of three children, born 1966, she was a graduate in Hospitality Management, BAA 1991, Toronto

Erin worked in the hotel and restaurant business in both Vancouver and Toronto.

She was diagnosed with ovarian cancer at thirty-one in February 1998.

All her life, Erin taught people by telling stories. When she was faced cancer she immediately began journalling about her experiences, treatments and emotions. She wrote as if she were speaking to the reader with honest, open and gut-wrenching reality. Her friends said "Erin was always a storyteller, outspoken, animated and funny." This time the story was about her and her journal writings are genuine and direct from her heart.

Alma C. Lightbody

Has degrees in Medical Technology, an MBA in Business and multiple certificates in Management, Holistic Health, and Shamanic Healing with the last twenty years focused on Energy Medicine. Alma worked closely with Erin as a wellness practitioner for three years and was asked by Erin to compile a book from her journals to pass on her story. Erin's journals are written with passion and inspiration, as she shares valuable and profound lessons and insights. Alma is proud to be the co-author in the production of this book.

What would Erin say?

- Our bodies talk to us and we don't know how to 'listen'
- Get to know yourself – don't wait
- Don't let doctors tell you nothing is wrong
- Nobody is going to cure you but you
- Do what you love, it's good for your immune system
- Find what your purpose in life is – mine is to teach others through my journals and book
- Learn to speak your truth
- Take one day at a time and enjoy every moment
- My Spirituality heightens every day
- Laughter is very important in healing
- I love my body – it is my temple and must be honoured
- Use your intuition to 'listen to your body'
- When someone bothers you it's often a mirror image of something you need to learn about yourself
- Soulfulness is truly what everything is all about
- When I ask you to respect my needs, please do so
- I feel comfortable about the afterlife; my soul will live on
- Pain is a physical manifestation of the growth of your soul
- Support groups should be filled with positive healing energy zipping around the room
- We must never assume the best place for a soul is among the living, for that may not be
- Rebirth-Review-Revise-Recycle-Redo-Begin again

We invite you to continue your experience with Erin through excerpts from her video at

www.MyWonderfulNightmare.com

About the videos

May 22, 2010

Tears are streaming down my face, but I'm not sad. Watching those 24 minutes of Erin's film have left me with an overwhelming feeling of hope, love, and thanks. Erin Higgins made her mark on me a long, long time ago. First, as my friend's big sister: dynamic, gregarious, self-confident, and sensitive all at the same time. And, she made me laugh. Her zany sense of humour just seemed to fit with mine (and many others, I suppose) and her laughter was absolutely infectious. I met Erin through Lara, who has been one of my best friends since the first moment we met at university. Erin was her older sister. In ways that I did not understand until after she was gone, Erin was not only Lara's big sister; she was my very dear friend too.

When I started journalism school, we were told the first day of our studies that our major project would consist of a mini-documentary that I suppose would demonstrate our journalistic abilities. We were to use all the skills we would learn throughout our training, and present a final work that we would each write, shoot, edit, and produce ourselves. I remember that first day thinking to myself: *I wonder what story is going to present itself that will be worthy of such dedication, work, creativity, passion, love, and energy.* I knew that whatever it would turn out to be, I would end up giving the topic as much of my love as I could to tell whatever story needed to be told. I was grateful for the challenge.

It took only a few months and I knew whom I wanted to interview: Erin Higgins.

I remember calling Erin and asking her if she had a story to tell. Little did I know that, by simply sitting down with her in her apartment, surrounded by tulips and photographs, art and books, all I would need to do is just listen. Erin would do the rest. It was a very special afternoon I spent with Erin that day, intimate and inspiring both at the same time. I simply asked the questions; Erin shared her story. She was a natural storyteller, her powerful presence as captivating as her boundless spirit. Erin was diagnosed with cancer but, for her, nothing was terminal about it. She was determined to spread her message: to help other people learn to listen to their bodies and become empowered by their own health. She was smart, insightful, generous, and kind. I felt almost selfish that there was little I could do for her, but offer her a diary in which to write about her life… and give her this documentary that would timelessly tell her tale. *But, would she like the film that I would produce? Would I tell her story in a way that would remain respectful and true to her? Would it be possible that I could assist in transmitting her message to the world?* Erin spoke and I listened. Now I wanted to make it possible for others to listen too. Erin had a voice, and I wanted to do all I could to make sure that it would be heard.

That was almost 10 years ago. I can't believe so much time has passed. A lot has changed since then, but one thing remains: Erin. When she was diagnosed with ovarian cancer, Erin fought (and fought she did) relentlessly for two years and nine months, leaving behind the lasting impression that she imprinted on everyone who had ever had the privilege of coming into contact with her. (I feel even extra blessed for having gotten to know her much more deeply during that one afternoon interview.) Now, all of these years later, I am living in Scandinavia and whenever I see a bouquet of tulips – be it at an open market in the spring, on a table in a little café, or growing freely in an expansive and colourful field – I think it's Erin's way of saying hello. There she is overlooking flowers at a market. There she is at a table in a café. There she is walking through a field. It would not be right for me to say that she is here "in" Sweden, for I know that wherever anyone is who has ever met and loved this amazing woman, Erin is right there with them too.

Two days ago, I found out that Erin's healing touch therapist, Alma Lightbody had a friend edit the hours of footage that I had left behind of my afternoon with Erin. Alma mailed me the short 3-part film, and asked me to view it. This took me by surprise, and I must admit that I was a bit scared. So many years had now passed since my interview with Erin, her devastating passing, the celebration of her life, and the showing of my short documentary at her funeral. I was not sure I was ready to face Erin's pain again. However, I thought about her the entire day. Was I ready to "go there" again? Did I want to bring up memories that were safely tucked away? However, I did want to help Alma and Erin's family by preserving a small glimpse of the all-consuming personality of this proud and dignified woman. Surely, I decided, I would find the time and the strength to watch this film and "visit" with Erin again.

I went to bed that night and had a very fitful sleep; I thought a lot about Erin and the pain that she had been through. Image after image flooded my mind of my dear Lara and her loving family who continue to miss Erin every single day of their lives. At one point, I sat straight up in my bed – 3 o'clock in the morning - awakened by an extremely vivid dream. There were no images that I remember, no colours, no forms. There was only one voice. It was Erin speaking to me again. She was calm and compelling, and she spoke to me as clearly as though she was sitting in the same room. Erin kept saying: *"Tell them to think of me, Karyn, and not my illness. Tell them to remember not my illness... Tell them just to remember me."*

And so, that was it. I got up out of bed and watched the film. And, I am so glad that I did. How delighted I am for the sensitive and thoughtful way in which Alma's friend Ronnie Novak (whom I've never even met) edited the sweeping passages of my heartfelt conversation with Erin all those years ago, linking together the main messages that Erin wanted the world to know, and captivating the very essence of her sparkling being. Best Friend, Big Sister, Loving Daughter, Cherished Kin... Erin touched the hearts of many. She was strong. She was kind. And, she taught us all to listen to our bodies, to trust our inner voice, to learn as much as we can, and to embrace whatever life throws our way. Through the power of video, the love of those she left behind, and the words of a woman determined and proud, Erin Higgins lives on.

And for that, I will be forever grateful.

"Tell them to remember not my illness... Tell them just to remember me."

~Karyn McGettigan

The videos are available at:

www.MyWonderfulNightmare.com